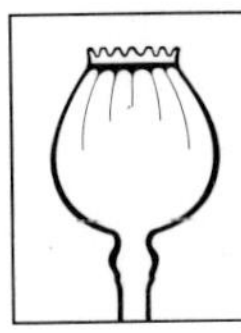

Current Topics in Anaesthesia

General Editors: Stanley A. Feldman
Cyril F. Scurr

1 Intravenous Anaesthetic Agents

Intravenous Anaesthetic Agents

John W. Dundee,
MD, PhD, FFA,RCS, MRCP
Professor of Anaesthetics
The Queen's University of Belfast, Northern Ireland

Edward Arnold

First published 1979
by Edward Arnold (Publishers) Ltd.
41 Bedford Square, London WC1B 3DQ
Reprinted 1979

British Library Cataloguing in Publication Data
Dundee, John Wharry
Intravenous anaesthetic agents. — (Current topics in anaesthesia).
1. Intravenous anaesthesia
I. Title II. Series
617′.962 RD85.16

ISBN 0-7131-4332-0

Text photoset in 10/11pt. Compugraphic Times by The Lavenham Press Ltd., Lavenham, Suffolk and printed in Great Britain by Unwin Brothers Ltd., The Gresham Press, Old Woking, Surrey.

General preface to series

The current rate of increase of scientific knowledge is such that it is recognized that '. . . ninety per cent of all the existing knowledge which can be drawn upon for the practice of medicine is less than 10 years old'.*

In an acute specialty, such as anaesthesia, failure to keep abreast of advances can seriously affect the standard of patient care. The need for continuing education is widely recognized and indeed it is mandatory in some countries.

However, due to the flood of new knowledge which grows in an exponential fashion greatly multiplying the pool of information every decade, the difficulty which presents itself is that of selecting and retrieving the information of immediate value and clinical relevance. This series has been produced in an effort to overcome this dilemma.

By producing a number of authoritative reviews the Current Topics Series has allowed the General Editors to select those in which it is felt there is a particular need for a digest of the large amount of literature, or for a clear statement of the relevance of new information.

By presenting these books in a concise form it should be possible to publish these reviews quickly. Careful selection of authors allows the presentation of mature clinical judgement on the relative importance of this new information.

The information will be clearly presented and, by emphasizing only key references and by avoiding an excess of specialist jargon, the books will, it is hoped, prove to be useful and succinct.

It has been our intention to avoid the difficulties of the large textbooks, with their inevitable prolonged gestation period, and to produce books with a wider appeal than the comprehensive, detailed, and highly specialized monographs. By this means we hope that the Current Topics in Anaesthesia Series will make a valuable contribution by meeting the demands of continuing education in anaesthesia.

Westminster Hospital
London

Stanley A. Feldman
Cyril F. Scurr

* Education and Training for the Professions.
Sir Frank Hartley, Wilkinson Lecture,
Delivered at Institute of Dental Surgery, 30.1.78
University of London Bulletin, May 1978, No. 45, p. 3.

Preface

This is not a textbook on intravenous anaesthetics, neither is it an updating supplement to the 1974 edition of *Intravenous Anaesthesia.* Rather, as the title conveys, it is intended to be a survey of what were considered to be topical items during the three months of its writing (January-March 1978).

The author has been engaged in the study of intravenous anaesthetics for over a quarter of a century and this has provided useful background knowledge against which to consider the current topics. To give these relevance in relation to established knowledge it has been necessary to include a brief survey of the present status of the barbiturates and eugenols. Such a review would have been impossible with althesin, as there is no established view on its place in anaesthesia; rather an attempt has been made to suggest a rational approach to its use to make the most of the many excellent qualities and to limit its dangers.

Most will agree that anaphylactoid reactions to intravenous anaesthetics is the major current talking point. This subject has been reviewed in depth by my colleague Richard Clarke in what is the longest chapter in this book. As one of the authors of a published report on a survey of 100 cases of sensitivity to intravenous anaesthetics, he has the necessary knowledge to put this subject into its true perspective. One hopes that this survey will help readers to clarify their views on hypersensitivity and be aware of this most dangerous aspect of the action of intravenous anaesthetics.

It is inevitable that a book of this nature reflects some of my personal current interests. This may partly explain the space devoted to ketamine. Ken Lilburn's collaboration in this has enabled me to draw on his experience of two years full-time research with this interesting drug. Some may feel that enough time and effort has already been given to 'taming' it and that it should join bromethol, vinesthene and ethylene. An apology is offered to those who feel that my knowledge of research in this field could have been put to better advantage.

This element of personal choice may be reflected in the inclusion of a lengthy discussion on the benzodiazepines and a briefer review on balanced techniques.

What of etomidate? To have omitted it or give it just brief mention may not have detracted from the value of the book to the average reader. However, there is no extensive review of it in the English language and the current one has given us an opportunity of comparing our findings with those of continental workers. Matthew Zacharias, who collaborated on this chapter, has undoubtedly more personal experience with etomidate than anyone in Britain and in the light of our finding it is hard to envisage a bright future for it.

Preface

There are three clinical fields in which there is much disagreement as to the place of intravenous anaesthetics. I have been fortunate to get the views of three experienced colleagues, on paediatrics (Sam Keilty), obstetrics (James Moore) and cardiac surgery (Ian Carson). Each of these has given his own views, rather than reviewing the literature and this should help clarify the position of intravenous drugs in the relevant fields.

A book on current topics must be written in a hurry and published before it is out of date. For this reason the bibliography has been kept to a minimum except in the major topics. It is an interesting experience to have a 'longhand-to-Editors' interval of about three months and this has not allowed time for rewriting or lengthy corrections. Such speed has only been possible with the cooperation of many colleagues and particularly the junior department staff who corrected tables, prepared diagrams, checked references etc. Above all an experienced typist, capable of reading my corrected manuscript and making sense of it has been an essential. To Noelle Collins I am particularly indebted for perfectly filling this role.

Belfast April 1978 John W. Dundee

Acknowledgements

I am grateful to the following authors and journals and publishers for permission to reproduce figures and tables: Dr A. Doenicke (Fig. 3.1), Dr A. Sutton (Table 4.1), Dr B. Kay (Fig. 6.5), Dr W. Lorenz (Fig. 8.2) and Dr J. Watkins (Fig. 8.3); *Canadian Anaesthetists' Society Journal* (Fig. 3.1), *Anaesthesia* (Fig. 3.2), *British Journal of Anaesthesia* (Figs. 6.5, 7.8 and 8.2), *British Journal of Clinical Pharmacology* (Fig. 7.5), *Acta anaesthesiologica Scandinavica* (Fig. 7.4), Excerpta Medica (Table 4.1), Academic Press (Fig. 8.3).

J.W.D.

Contents

Glossary of drugs

Generic Names		Proprietary names*
UK	Others	
Alphadolone/Alphaxalone	CT1341	Althesin, Alfatésine
Amylobarbitone	Amobarbital	AMYTAL, Intrased, Isonal, Novamobarb, Amaytalily, Dormytal, Eunoctal
Buthalitone		Baytinal, Transithal, Ulbreval
Butobarbitone		SONERYL, Butisal, Interbarb, Metubal
Chlormethiazole	S.C.T.Z.	Heminevrin
Chlorpromazine		LARGACTIL, THORAZINE, Chlor-Promanyl, Chlorprom-Ez-Etz, Elmarine, Onazine, Promosol, Hibanul, Megaphen
Diazepam		Valium, Vivol, Apaurin, Eridan, Lembrol, Noan, Setonil, Tranimul, Vatran
Doxapram		DOPRAM, Doxapril, Stimulexin
Droperidol		INAPSINE, Droleptan
Fentanyl		Sublimaze
Flurazepam		Dalmane
Gamma-Hydroxybutyrate	Gamma-OH	
Hexobarbitone	Hexobarbital	EVIPAL, Evipan, Cyclonal, Hexenol, ENa, Oevipana-Sodico, Oulopan-Natrium
Hydroxydione		Viadril, Presuren
Hyoscine	Scopolamine	Buscpan, Kwells, Pamine, Isopto-Hyoscine
Fentanyl/droperidol	Innovar	Thalamonal
Ketamine		KETALAR, Ketaject
Levorphanol	Levorphan	DROMORAN, Levo-Dromoran
Lorazepam		Ativan, Larpose
Medazepam		Nobrium
Mephenesin		MYANESIN, Tolserol, Dioloxol, Sinan, Tolyspaz
Methohexitone	Methohexital	BRIETAL, Brevimytal, Brevital
Nalorphine		NALLINE, Lethidrone, Norfin
Neostigmine		PROSTIGMIN
Nitrazepam		Megadon, Mogadon, Nitretamine
Oxazepam		SERAX, Adumbran, Limbial Praxiten, Serenid-D, Seresta
Pentobarbitone	Pentobarbital	NEMBUTAL, Butylone, Hypnol, Hypnotal, Ibatal, Novopentobarb, Nova-Rectal, Pental, Pentanca, Pentogen, Somnotol
Pethidine	Meperidine Isonipecaine	DEMEROL, Phytadon, Dolantal, Dolantin, Mefedina
Phenoperidine		OPERIDINE
Promethazine		PHENERGAN, Histantil, Atosil
Propanidid	FBA 1420	EPONTOL, Fabontal
Quinalbarbitone	Secobarbital	SECONAL, Novosecobarb, S.C.B. Tal, Secaps, Secocaps, Secogen, Secotaps, Hyptrol, Sedonal, Seotal, Tuisec
Suxamethonium	Succinylcholine	ANECTINE, Brevidil, 'M', Quelicin, Scoline, Sucostrin, Sux-Cert
Thialbarbitone	Thialbarbital	KEMITHAL, Kemithene
Thiobutobarbitone		Inactin, Inaktin
	Thioethanyl	Venesetic
Thiopentone	Thiopental Thionembutal	PENTOTHAL, INTRAVAL, Trapanal Nesdonal, Penthiobarbital Sodique, Farmotal, Pentothal Natricum, Pentothal Sodico, Hipnopento

*The trade names in capitals are the most widely used.

1

Classification of intravenous anaesthetics

Although this book includes drugs other than those used principally to produce intravenous anaesthesia, it is useful to consider the manner in which the intravenous anaesthetic agents have been classified because it reveals an interdependence of three pharmacological activities:

1. Pharmacokinetics.
2. Chemical structure.
3. Clinical acceptability

Duration of action

The terms 'ultra-short-acting' and 'short-acting' are often applied indiscriminately to intravenous anaesthetics. These terms are not only confusing but may also be misleading and may have serious consequences for those not aware of the pharmacokinetics of the drugs. 'Ultra-short-acting' and 'short-acting' should be reserved for drugs which are rapidly broken down in the body and from which rapid recovery is not dependent on redistribution to non-nervous tissues. On this basis the terms are only applicable to:

Ultra-short-acting	propanidid (Epontol, Fabontal)
Short-acting	Althesin (Alfatesine, CT 1341)

In contrast with these truly short acting drugs, the termination of action of intravenous barbiturate (thiobarbiturate or methylbarbiturate) and the return of consciousness occur when there is a large amount of active drug remaining in the body. There is therefore always the possibility that these patients may relapse into unconsciousness if left undisturbed, especially if drugs given in the early postoperative period themselves lead to some depression of consciousness.

Onset of action

It is desirable for induction agents to have a rapid onset of action. Ideally, in adequate doses they should produce sleep in one arm–brain circulation time, so that dosage can be accurately titrated against the patient's requirements. Drugs with a slow onset of action are essentially basal hypnotics.

In general, drugs with a rapid onset of action have a shorter duration of action than more slowly acting compounds. The primary induction agents (rapidly acting) also produce fewer side effects — excluding immediate cardiovascular and respiratory depression — than the slower acting (basal hypnotic) drugs. These latter drugs should be used only when specifically indicated. The following classification separates the various groups of drugs according to the rate of onset and their chemical constituents, rather than according to their duration of action (the more usual but less appropriate classification).

Rapidly acting

Induction agents:	thiobarbiturates, methylbarbiturates eugenols Althesin (steroid) etomidate sulphate (imidazole)

Slower acting

Basal hypnotics:	phencyclidines (ketamine) tranquillizers (diazepam, etc.) neuroleptic drug combinations and intravenous analgesics others: sodium oxybutyrate (Gamma-OH), chlormethiazole (Heminevrin), barbiturates

It should be noted that the barbiturates (such as pentobarbitone), which are generally employed as oral hypnotics, can be used intravenously — when they will have a moderately rapid onset of action.

Barbiturates

In addition to the above, these rapidly acting drugs can be classified either according to their chemistry or according to their clinical acceptability.

Chemistry (see Table 2.1)

Thiobarbiturates	thiopentone, thiamylal, thiobutobarbitone, buthalitone*, methitural*, thialbarbitone
Methylbarbiturates	hexobarbitone*, methohexitone, enibomal (Narkotal)

Clinical acceptability

Very satisfactory	equally acceptable	thiopentone, thiamylal, thiobutobarbitone, thialbarbitone
Unsatisfactory	too high an incidence of side effects	buthalitone*, methitural*, hexobarbitone*
Compromise	unique advantages, side effects	methohexitone, enibomal (Narkotal)

*These have been withdrawn from clinical use because of side effects.

Reference

Dundee, J. W. (1975). Classification of intravenous anaesthetics. In: *Recent Progress in Anaesthesiology and Resuscitation,* Proceedings of the IV European Congress of Anaesthesiology, Madrid, 5—11 September 1974, pp. 77—8. Ed. by A. Arias, R. Llaurado, M. A. Nalda and J. N. Lunn. Excerpta Medica, Amsterdam and Oxford; American Elsevier, New York.

2

The present status of the barbiturates

Barbiturates were the first successful intravenous anaesthetics and they remain the most popular anaesthetic induction agents. It is helpful to look at the reasons for their early acceptance and continuing clinical popularity — which has been achieved in spite of dangerous and occasionally lethal complications — since these drugs are the standards against which all new intravenous drugs are judged.

It has to be appreciated that, historically, not only were the intravenous barbiturates a new type of drug but also a completely new concept, viz. loss of consciousness induced by agents given intravenously. Perhaps just as important was the fact that it coincided with the development of the technique of 'balanced' anaesthesia — which restricted the use of the intravenous barbiturates to the production of hypnosis and thus limited the early abuse which followed their introduction. This, in fact, also resulted in the use of safe doses by the avoidance of the toxicity of large cumulative doses.

Barbiturates

Four chemical groups of barbiturates have been used, and Table 2.1 shows the relationship of the 1 and 2 position side chains to their group characteristics when given intravenously. The methyl thiobarbiturates are not used clinically and are included in the Table solely for the sake of completeness.

In practice, the (oxy)barbiturates are used mainly as night-time hypnotics adminstered by mouth. Occasionally they are used in psychiatric practice in small doses as basal sedatives. The absence, in Britain, of a commercially available stable solution of any of these drugs has hampered their use as a preanaesthetic medication, an indication for which they are widely employed in North America. The very active Campaign for the Use and Restriction of Barbiturates (CURB) propaganda of 1976—1977 was aimed at reducing the overprescribing of barbiturates as sedatives and reducing the incidence of dependence on these drugs. This is not likely to have much effect on their very limited use in the preoperative period, although it may have lessened the incidence of their prescription as a night sedative. However, in general, the benzodiazepines (diazepam, nitrazepam and, more recently, lorazepam) are widely considered to be the drugs of choice for patient sedation on the night before operation.

There is available a preparation containing pentobarbitone sodium 60

Table 2.1 Relationship of chemical grouping to clinical action of barbiturates

H^+

Pyrimidine derivative

Keto form ⇌ Enol form

Cyclical ureide of malonic acid

Group	Substituents position 1	Substituents position 2	Group characteristics when given intravenously
(Oxy)barbiturates	H	O	Delay in onset of action, degree depending on 5 and 5′ side chains. Useful as basal hypnotics. Prolonged action
Methyl barbiturates	CH_3	O	Usually rapidly acting with fairly rapid recovery. High incidence of excitatory phenomena
Thiobarbiturates	H	S	Rapidly acting, usually smooth onset of sleep and fairly prompt recovery
Methyl thiobarbiturates	CH_3	S	Rapid onset of action and very rapid recovery but with so high an incidence of excitatory phenomena as to preclude use in clinical practice

mg/ml (Nembutal) made up with propylene glycol (20 per cent v/v) and alcohol (10 per cent v/v). Although intended as a veterinary preparation, it has been used as a sedative in intensive care work and, to a lesser extent, for premedication. This solution causes an unacceptably high incidence of persistent pain at the i.m. injection site (which does not occur with freshly prepared aqueous solutions). Although it has a greater soporific effect than the same dose of pentobarbitone given by mouth, it has a poor anxiolytic action and is inferior to diazepam as a premedicant.

Methylbarbiturates

Amylobarbitone and pentobarbitone were the earliest barbiturates to be used as intravenous anaesthetics. They were later replaced by hexobarbitone (Evipan, Evipal), a methylated barbiturate. The success of this drug was not due to the more rapid recovery but rather to the quicker onset of action so that the dose could be more easily titrated against the needs of the patient. Hexobarbitone caused a high incidence of excitatory effects (spontaneous involuntary muscle movement and/or tremor).

Another methylbarbiturate, methohexitone, is popular as an induction agent, particularly for outpatients. It is two to three times more potent than thiopentone and is used in a 1—2 per cent solution. It has a lower tissue toxicity than thiopentone whether following subcutaneous or intra-arterial injection. This may be due to the less concentrated solution used or it may be associated with the absence of the sulphur atom. Induction of anaesthesia with methohexitone is followed by an appreciable incidence of extraneous muscle movements although these are less marked than with hexobarbitone. The factors which influence the frequency and severity of these movements have been studied in detail and it has been shown that both the total dose of drug and the speed of injection affect the incidence and severity of the muscle movements. The incidence is reduced by the use of an opiate premedication (or the administration of fentanyl immediately before the induction of anaesthesia) but increased by the preoperative use of promethazine or hyoscine (Table 2.2). Respiratory complications (cough and hiccough) are often troublesome with methohexitone but can be minimized by injecting the drug slowly and by using a small total dose.

Table 2.2. Percentage incidence of excitatory phenomena (spontaneous involuntary muscle movement, hypertonus or tremor) following equivalent doses of thiopentone and methohexitone given after different premedicants

Preanaesthetic medication	Thiopentone 4 mg·kg^{-1}	Methohexitone 1.6 mg·kg^{-1}
Atropine or nil	4	17
Hyoscine	18	46
Promethazine	25	70
Pethidine	4	7
Pethidine—hyoscine	6	25
Promethazine—hyoscine	46	87

Atropine premedication is also helpful in this respect. Another disadvantage of methohexitone is the sensation of pain on injection but figures as to its frequency or severity vary. Methohexitone is also more likely to induce epileptiform convulsions in susceptible patients than the other intravenous induction agents.

It is surprising that, despite these disadvantages and the fact that early claims concerning its lesser cardiovascular toxicity have not been confirmed, methohexitone continues to be used and is considered by many to be the induction agent of choice in certain situations (Whitwam, 1976). One of these is when early ambulation and a rapid turnover of patients are required; here the relatively rapid recovery which occurs after methohexitone, as compared with other intravenous anaesthetics, is the reason for its popularity.

Although early reports claimed that recovery was significantly shorter than after equivalent doses of thiopentone, it was hard to be sure if this was a true finding or only an illusion (because of the problems involved in assessing true recovery times). Objective evidence in support of this rapid recovery was provided by Carson, Graham and Dundee (1975) who also found a more rapid recovery after methohexitone than after Althesin.

Despite early claims that methohexitone is inactivated more rapidly in the body than thiopentone, it has been generally assumed that all intravenous barbiturates have a similar pharmacokinetic profile; i.e. rapid redistribution to non-nervous tissue with ultimate location of large amounts in body fat and a slow rate of metabolism. Qualitative differences between drugs are attributed principally to differences in lipid solubility rather than to metabolism. However, Breimer (1976), using sensitive chromatographic methods of measurement, has recently confirmed the more rapid metabolism of methohexitone which was found to have the relatively short half-life of 70—125 minutes. With this rapid metabolism there are smaller amounts of drug available for storage in fat and for eventual release into the blood. This work provides scientific evidence to justify the use of methohexitone in circumstances where a rapid return of consciousness is desired.

Whitwam (1976) has judged methohexitone against his criteria for the ideal induction agent and concludes a survey of its advantages and disadvantages by stating that 'methohexitone is the best drug currently available for the routine induction of anaesthesia by the intravenous route'. It is hard to disagree with his arguments if one accepts the overriding importance of an early recovery of complete consciousness. Furthermore, one would hesitate in recommending its use in large doses as sole agent even for minor procedures as the unpleasant sight of the patient sitting up in bed and periodically hiccoughing during recovery, or the occasional occurrence of severe spontaneous muscle movement, must be considered. Nevertheless, 20 years after its introduction, methohexitone is the only intravenous barbiturate which offers a serious challenge to thiopentone. In Chapter 1 it is classified as a barbiturate whose 'advantages outweigh its disadvantages' and this would seem to be an apt description.

Thiobarbiturates

Six thiobarbiturates have been used extensively in clinical anaesthesia and two of these (buthalitone and methitural) caused such a high incidence of complications on induction that they are no longer used. Methitural embraced an interesting concept in its formulation by including a sulphur atom in a thioethyl side chain in the hope that this would accelerate its breakdown and at the same time liberate methionine which would protect the liver from the toxic effects of the barbiturates. It is perhaps timely to recall that pharmacologists and anaesthetists were at one time concerned about the potential hepatotoxic effects of intravenous anaesthetics. We are acutely aware of the potential dangers of inhalational agents in this respect but should not forget that large doses of intravenous agents may be equally toxic. This is discussed later in relation to total intravenous anaesthesia (Chapter 11).

Four thiobarbiturates are acceptable as induction agents but thiopentone is by far the most popular of these. Thiamylal is slightly more potent than thiopentone (estimated as 1.1 : 1.0), but otherwise the two drugs are clinically indistinguishable. Thiamylal is not commercially available in Britain. Thiobutobarbitone is only about 70 per cent as potent as thiopentone (w/w); it is commercially available in parts of continental Europe under the trade name of Inactin (Inaktin). Thialbarbitone is only half as potent as thiopentone, and for some years it was used in 5 and 10 per cent solutions which were clinically equivalent to 2.5 and 5 per cent thiopentone. These high concentrations created solubility problems and caused an increased risk should accidental arterial injection occur. Another interesting point about thialbarbitone (Kemithal) was its distinct odour which pervaded the hands of its users for several days. At the time of writing it is not commercially available in Britain but is still used in South America. Thialbarbitone was the only drug in this series which was synthesized and evaluated in Britain.

One could readily dismiss thiopentone in this chapter by saying that it is the world's most popular induction agent and that familiarity with its use has contributed to its overall safety. It is by no means a perfect intravenous anaesthetic, yet we have learned to live with its failings. At a time when much interest is being shown in new intravenous induction agents, it is the yardstick against which these should be judged (Table 2.3).

Like its immediate predecessor, hexobarbitone, it causes sleep in one arm—brain circulation time. However, in contrast to hexobarbitone which caused an unacceptably high incidence of involuntary movements, thiopentone usually produces a smooth, quiet induction. In some patients there may be minor limb movements but these are not troublesome. They occur more frequently after the rapid injection of large doses of drug and, like methohexitone, their incidence and severity are affected by the nature of the premedication, being reduced by opiates and increased by phenothiazines such as promethazine, by hyoscine or other non-analgesic drugs. The smoothness of induction by thiopentone, as compared with methohexitone, is shown in Table 2.2, which is a comparison of the incidence of excitatory effects found in several very large series of patients following the administration of equivalent doses of the two induction agents. Laryngospasm was once considered to be a dangerous complication of thiopentone but this has lost its terrors since suxamethonium became available. However, this complication is rarely encountered in adequately atropinized patients unless there has been a minor degree of regurgitation of gastric contents or a direct irritation to the larynx.

Much has been written about the absence of analgesic action of thiopentone (an antanalgesic activity has even been ascribed to it). There appears to be much confusion as to what this term implies. Perhaps this is due to the word 'antanalgesic' which perhaps might be better replaced by 'hyperalgesia' — i.e. the increased appreciation of a painful stimulus. Subnarcotic doses of thiopentone increase the patient's sensitivity to somatic pain and

Table 2.3 The advantages and disadvantages of thiopentone

	Advantages	Disadvantages
Physical properties	Soluble in water Easily injectable solution No pain on injection	Not stable in solution Highly alkaline solution Irritant on subcutaneous or arterial injection
Induction	Rapidly acting Consistent effect Smooth induction Low incidence of hypersensitivity reactions Minimal cardiovascular and respiratory depression in small doses No interference with action of neuromuscular blocking drugs	Antanalgesic action in small doses No analgesic action, even in large doses Unpredictable response to painful stimuli Potential hazard of laryngospasm Unfit patients show an exaggerated response to its depressant effect
Anaesthesia	Adequate duration of induction dose to allow gaseous or volatile supplementation Can be given intermittently	Not a 'sole anaesthetic' Readily crosses placental barrier Cumulative effect on intermittent injection Potential hepatotoxic effects of large doses
Recovery	Usually smooth No emetic effects	Due to redistribution rather than detoxication Delay in return of full mental faculties Prolonged sensitivity to pain after large doses Not suitable for unaccompanied outpatients

this state of antanalgesia, which is associated with a low brain concentration of thiopentone, occurs during induction and during recovery from large doses of the drug. It appears to apply only to the pain of deep pressure (such as that produced by pressure on the tibia) since small doses of thiopentone have been shown to reduce the ability to appreciate a painful stimulus applied directly to the skin. Small doses of thiopentone appear to antagonize the analgesia produced by nitrous oxide and pethidine in experimental situations. This seems to contradict the established clinical experience that the addition of nitrous oxide enhances the action of thiopentone; in fact, the nitrous oxide—oxygen administered is used to compensate for the missing analgesic component in thiopentone anaesthesia. As long ago as 1938, Organe and Broad demonstrated that much smaller doses of thiopentone were required to produce satisfactory anaesthesia when the drug was injected intermittently than when nitrous oxide was also being administered.

Even large doses of thiopentone appear to be devoid of a specific analgesic action. With the barbiturates, perhaps more than any other drugs used widely in anaesthesia, the clinical level of anaesthesia is related to the intensity of the surgical stimulus as well as to the degree of cerebral depression. After thiopentone, an undisturbed patient, with depressed respiration and abdominal and masseteric relaxation, may give a picture of moderately deep surgical anaesthesia, but on application of a surgical stimulus the respiration is stimulated, relaxation lost and there may be reflex movement of a limb. If this patient is given sufficient thiopentone to produce surgical anaesthesia in the presence of strong stimulation, a dangerous degree of respiratory depression and prolonged unconsciousness may occur when the stimulation ceases.

While the analgesic drugs will reduce the dose of thiopentone required to produce surgical anaesthesia, because they also depress respiration and most are long acting, a similar state can be produced to an excessive dose of thiopentone, especially if a large dose of analgesic is given too near to the end of the operation. With the use of nitrous oxide—oxygen to supplement thiopentone it is possible to produce a satisfactory pattern of anaesthesia without excessive dosage of thiopentone or analgesics and without causing dangerous and prolonged depression of vital functions.

Although much emphasis has been placed on the cardiovascular and respiratory depressant effects of thiopentone, in practice these are minimal in fit patients. Perhaps it is hoping for too much to find a drug which will not produce these untoward effects in ill patients, but in practice the slow administration of small doses of thiopentone are well tolerated by most patients. The correction of hypovolaemia and the avoidance of opiate or phenothiazine premedication, together with preoxygenation, can further increase the safety of this procedure.

Many claims have been made for the lesser cardiovascular toxicity of the newer intravenous anaesthetics in poor-risk patients. In general, significant advantages have not been substantiated for these agents. Lyons and Clarke (1972), Lyons, Clarke and Dundee (1974) and Clarke and Lyons (1977) gave equivalent doses of several intravenous induction agents to heavily pre-medicated patients prior to cardiac surgery. Five minutes after injection a similar fall in blood pressure was found after thiopentone 4 $mg{\cdot}kg^{-1}$, methohexitone 1.5 $mg{\cdot}kg^{-1}$, propanidid 4 $mg{\cdot}kg^{-1}$, Althesin 0·05 $\mu l{\cdot}kg^{-1}$, diazepam 0·36 $mg{\cdot}kg^{-1}$ and flunitrazepam 0.032 $mg{\cdot}kg^{-1}$. This fall occurred most rapidly with propanidid and most slowly with the two benzodiazepines. Methohexitone caused the highest incidence of tachycardia.

While it is feasible to give thiopentone by intermittent injection, this is not recommended except in short procedures. Large doses produce enzyme changes which are consistent with liver dysfunction and should be avoided. The potential of 'total intravenous anaesthesia' as a means of eliminating theatre pollution is attractive but, for reasons which are discussed fully in Chapter 11, thiopentone and similar drugs are not recommended for this purpose.

It has been fairly well established that recovery from thiopentone is due to redistribution in the body rather than to rapid detoxication, although drug metabolism by liver mitochondria is probably more important than originally envisaged (Saidman and Eger, 1966). Even allowing for the effects of metabolism, there is no justification for considering thiopentone to be an ultra-short-acting drug. A large amount of unmetabolized drug remains in the body for at least 12 hours after its administration and this may potentiate the action of alcohol or other barbiturates taken postoperatively. Diazepam and opiate narcotics can also have an exaggerated depressant effect if taken in the early postoperative period. The use of thiopentone to anaesthetize unaccompanied outpatients is unjustified and patients must be told to avoid tasks requiring fine discrimination or thought for the remainder of the day following such an anaesthetic.

A family or personal history of acute intermittent porphyria is the only absolute contraindication to the use of thiopentone. An acute exacerbation of the disease is not induced every time one gives the drug (Ward, 1965) but, since an acute attack carries about a 1 in 10 risk of a fatal outcome, clearly there is no justification for its administration to a known (or even suspected) porphyric.

Acute hypersensitivity reactions to intravenous anaesthetics are being reported with increasing frequency, and this topic is reviewed more fully in Chapter 8. While most reports concern Althesin, there appears to be an increasing incidence following thiopentone which cannot be explained solely by more consistent observation and reporting. It would appear to reflect an absolute increase in these complications (Dundee, 1976; Clarke, Fee and Dundee, 1977). Although it does not occur as commonly as reported following Althesin, one distinct feature of acute hypersensitivity reactions to thiopentone is the greater likelihood of a fatal outcome as compared with that following the steroid anaesthetic.

At one time it was stated dogmatically that one would have to look to non-barbiturates for advances in intravenous anaesthesia. Barbiturates have certain undesirable actions which are common to all; for example, antanalgesia, dose-related cardiovascular depression, irritant (alkaline) solutions, recovery due to redistribution rather than rapid detoxication. They would appear to be drugs which combine a depressant and stimulant action to varying degrees. While side chain changes have modified the severity and incidence of induction complications, they have not affected the basic barbiturate-type pharmacokinetics. Even the recent demonstration of a more rapid metabolism of methohexitone than had been expected still does not alter the fact that it is not a short-acting drug. Nevertheless, once its dangers and limitations are appreciated, the safety record of thiopentone can have few rivals in medicine. The list of advantages of thiopentone given in Table 2.3 can be equalled only by Althesin (which regrettably fails on the high incidence of hypersensitivity reactions Chapter 8). It would appear that we are unlikely to find a barbiturate which will prove to have substantial advantages over thiopentone, and this has encouraged research into the pharmacology of non-barbiturate induction agents.

Before leaving the topic, it is important to note that many of our current techniques of general anaesthesia, which include an intravenous induction are based on the expected duration of action of clinical doses of thiopentone. This was demonstrated when propanidid was experimentally substituted for thiopentone without any alteration in the general induction sequence: as a result of its short action there were many patients who recalled tracheal intubation, or wakened during suxamethonium paralysis; similarly, there were difficulties in inducing anaesthesia with the slowly acting volatile anaesthetics such as trichloroethylene and methoxyflurane (Penthrane) when the effects of the propanidid had worn off. Furthermore, one recalls the often disastrous falls in blood pressure which followed attempts to prolong the action of propanidid by increasing the dosage. Clinical anaesthetists have had over 30 years of cumulative experience of balanced techniques of anaesthesia based on both the known potency and the expected duration of action of thiopentone. Only a drug with a very obvious and substantial advantage will displace it from clinical use.

References

Breimer, D. D. (1976). Pharmacokinetics of methohexitone following intravenous infusion in humans. *British Journal of Anaesthesia* **48,** 643—9.

Carson, I. W., Graham, J. and Dundee, J. W. (1975). Clinical studies of induction agents. XLIII: Recovery from Althesin — a comparative study with thiopentone and methohexitone. *British Journal of Anaesthesia* **47,** 358—64.

Clarke, R. S. J., Fee, J. P. H. and Dundee, J. W. (1977). Factors predisposing to hypersensitivity reactions to intravenous anaesthetics. *Proceedings of the Royal Society of Medicine* **70,** 782—4.

Clarke, R. S. J. and Lyons, S. M. (1977). Diazepam and flunitrazepam as induction agents for cardiac surgical operations. *Acta anaesthesiologica Scandinavica* **4,** 282—92.

Dundee, J. W. (1976). Hypersensitivity to intravenous anaesthetics. *British Journal of Anaesthesia* **48,** 57—8.

Lyons, S. M. and Clarke, R. S. J. (1972). A comparison of different drugs for anaesthesia in cardiac surgical patients. *British Journal of Anaesthesia* **44,** 575—83.

Lyons, S. M., Clarke, R. S. J. and Dundee, J. W. (1974). Some cardiovascular and respiratory effects of four non-barbiturate anaesthetic induction agents. *European Journal of Clinical Pharmacology* **7,** 275—9.

Organe, G. S. W. and Broad, R. J. B. (1938). Pentothal with nitrous oxide and oxygen. *Lancet* **ii,** 1170—2.

Saidman, L. J. and Eger, E. I., II (1966). The effect of thiopental metabolism on duration of anesthesia. *Anesthesiology* **27,** 118—26.

Ward, R. J. (1965). Porphyria and its relation to anesthesia. *Anesthesiology* **26,** 212—15.

Whitwam, J. G. (1976). Methohexitone. *British Journal of Anaesthesia* **48,** 617—19.

3

The present position of the eugenols

The eugenols, so called because they are derived from oil of cloves, were the first drugs to offer any serious competition to the barbiturates as intravenous anaesthetics. Three of them have been used clinically and one, propanidid, still has a limited use in certain situations.

Like the barbiturates, this group of drugs has certain group characteristics (Table 3.1). In order to overcome their insolubility in water, solubilizing agents are used in the commercially available form of propanidid (Epontol, Fabontal) and these produce a viscid solution which necessitates the use of large needles. This can be a disadvantage, especially in children. However, the solution is miscible with water, which not only makes injection easier but also reduces the incidence of venous thrombosis. The difficulty of injecting a viscid solution rapidly can give the impression that propanidid takes slightly longer to exert an anaesthetic action than the barbiturates, but this is not substantiated at equal injection rates.

Table 3.1 Group characteristics of the intravenous eugenols

1. Insoluble in water
2. Rapidly acting
3. Initial respiratory stimulant action
4. Prolong the action of depolarizing myoneural blocking drugs
5. Side effects related to dosage and rate of injection
6. Rapid recovery due to detoxication

The feature which distinguishes the eugenols from all other available intravenous anaesthetics is the rapidity of complete recovery. Although, of necessity, a drug which is given intravenously will be redistributed in the body, the completeness of the early recovery is due to its rapid destruction by plasma cholinesterase to an acid metabolite with no anaesthetic properties. An interesting phenomenon is the effect of propanidid on the rate of its own metabolism; blood levels fall off more sharply after a rapid injection (and hence high peak concentration) than after slow injection, due to the higher concentration of substrate achieved for the enzymatic hydrolysis. On this basis, attempts to produce a longer period of sleep by giving larger doses are likely to be self-defeating, serving only to increase its toxicity.

The fact that propanidid is broken down by plasma cholinesterase means that patients with low serum levels of this enzyme could be expected to sleep longer after propanidid. This has, in fact, been demonstrated by electroencephalography (Doenicke *et al.*, 1968) and in these patients redistribution would be expected to play a major part in recovery. Except after prolonged intermittent administration of propanidid, this delay in breakdown is unlikely to be clinically apparent. Infusions of procaine, which would compete with the propanidid for the plasma cholinesterase, might also be expected to prolong the action of propanidid.

It is important to realize the full implications of the more rapid recovery from propanidid as compared with equivalent doses of the barbiturates. Doenicke and his colleagues in Munich have made intensive efforts to quantify the recovery from the drug by electroencephalography. In a series of papers (Doenicke and Kugler, 1965; Doenicke *et al.*, 1966; Doenicke, Kugler and Laub, 1967) it has been clearly demonstrated that not only is there a more rapid recovery of awake EEG activity than after thiopentone, hexobarbitone, thiobutobarbitone or methohexitone, but that there is also less tendency for the return of EEG evidence of sleep periods during the subsequent hours. The depth of sleep was assessed by integration of the amplitude of the encephalogram (Fig. 3.1), and the phases of sleepiness stand out clearly in the postoperative period. They also showed that 12 hours after methohexitone and the longer-acting drugs, the effects of half a litre of beer were potentiated, whereas after propanidid there were only the usual mild symptoms. Kreuscher (1955) also studied alertness for street traffic (Strassenverkehrstuchtigkeit) and concluded that 25 minutes after propanidid 500 mg a patient had regained his control level of response in a busy street.

This obviously has implications in the outpatient situation where alcohol may be used as a 'domestic analgesic'. Similarly, the taking of diazepam or other drugs is more likely to produce an exaggerated effect after barbiturates than after propanidid. However, too early recovery can occasionally lead to some restlessness, but this is not a major problem. It could perhaps account for the higher incidence of nausea and vomiting which occurs when propanidid is used for induction for minor operations as compared with similar patients given a barbiturate. This latter feature can be an undesirable side effect of its use in dental anaesthesia (Goldman and Kennedy, 1964).

It has been proved conclusively in several clinical studies that the average duration of apnoea and of respiratory depression following 50 mg suxamethonium is significantly longer when propanidid is given than when anaesthesia is induced with thiopentone or methohexitone. This is most likely to be due to the fact that the breakdown of both propanidid and suxamethonium is dependent on the same enzyme. This enzyme is inhibited temporarily by a high concentration of propanidid and it seems likely that the inhibition is involved in the more prolonged action of suxamethonium (Clarke, 1974).

Despite this established fact, in clinical practice one will often encounter patients in whom apnoea following thiopentone—suxamethonium is longer than that in similar patients having propanidid—suxamethonium. The

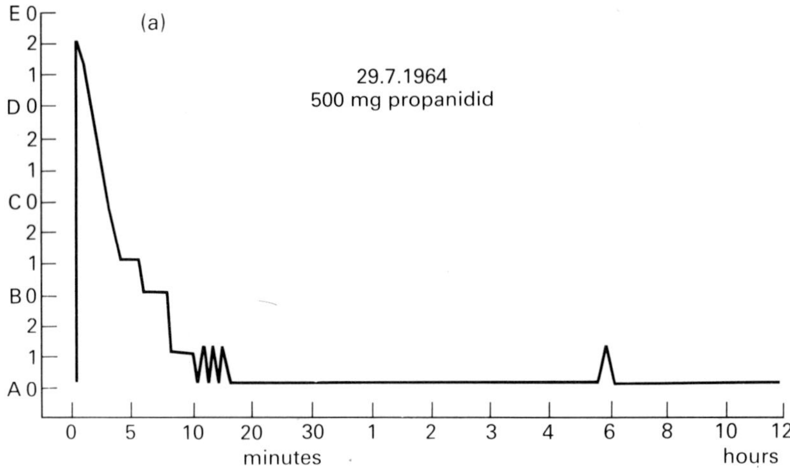

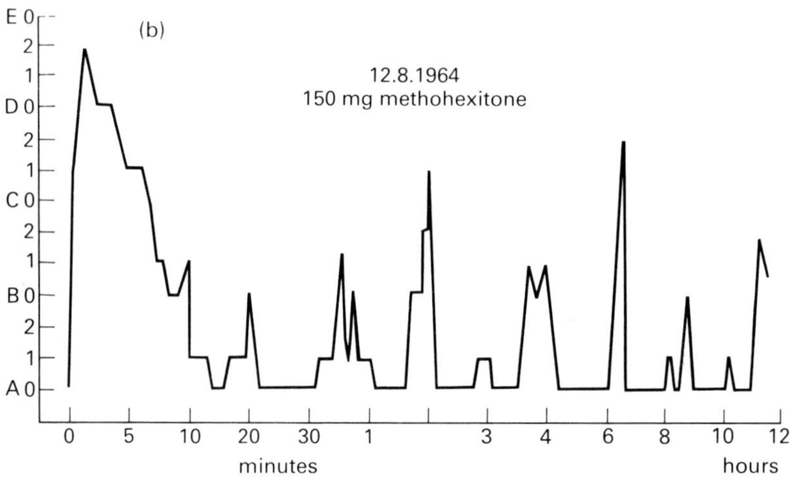

Fig. 3.1 Depth of sleep assessed from the electroencephalographic tracing according to Loomis' classification (ranging from A: very light sleep, to E: deep sleep), during and after (a) propanidid 500 mg and (b) methohexitone 150 mg. (From Doenicke, Kugler and Laub, 1967.)

reason for this may be explained by Fig. 3.2, which is based on the findings of Clarke, Dundee and Hamilton (1967). They measured the duration of apnoea and respiratory depression following 50 mg suxamethonium in three groups, each of 200 patients, induced with either thiopentone (average 5.2 $mg \cdot kg^{-1}$), methohexitone (average 1.6 $mg \cdot kg^{-1}$) or propanidid (average 6 $mg \cdot kg^{-1}$), with the results shown in Table 3.2. However, these figures tend to

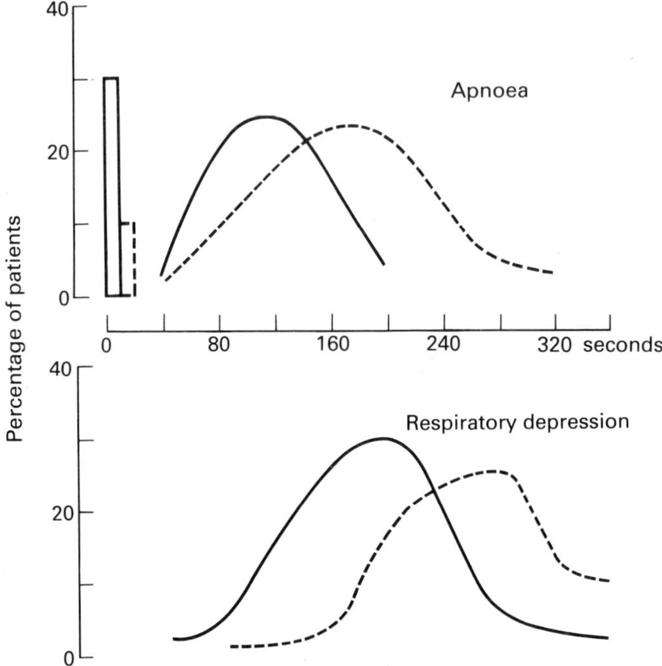

Fig. 3.2 Distribution of the duration of apnoea and respiratory depression in patients induced with a barbiturate (solid line) or propanidid (dashed line). (Free hand drawing of findings of Clarke, Dundee and Hamilton, 1967.)

conceal the wide scatter of individual readings. When the data obtained in the propanidid series are compared with the pooled barbiturate series, it will seem that there is quite an overlap, so that one is unlikely to notice this effect in clinical practice.

The use of propanidid—suxamethonium sequence can cause problems which the author recalls vividly from the early days of the clinical investiga-

Table 3.2 Average duration and range (seconds) of apnoea and respiratory depression after 50 mg suxamethonium in unselected groups of patients

	Thiopentone	Methohexitone	Propanidid
Apnoea			
Average duration	187 ± 9	205 ± 8	326 ± 11
Range	0—150	0—480	55—720
Respiratory depression			
Average duration	321 ± 21	321 ± 14	459 ± 31
Range	90—940	90—480	180—940

From Clarke, Dundee and Hamilton (1967)

tions of this induction agent. It was not unreasonable to expect that this drug would be of great use in endoscopies, particularly on outpatients. A short trial of propanidid—suxamethonium for bronchoscopy revealed an appreciable number of patients who not only awakened while the bronchoscope was still *in situ* but, equally distressing, found themselves awake and partially paralysed. The apprehension which this caused was understandable, particularly amongst the patients awaiting endoscopy!

However, propanidid still has much to offer for outpatient anaesthesia. It is the only truly 'ultra-short-acting' intravenous anaesthetic, although one would hesitate to recommend that the patient go home unaccompanied after its use. Furthermore, it does not have the antanalgesic action of thiopentone and is therefore useful as sole agent for short procedures. Its brevity of action necessitates rapid operation techniques and all preparations for surgery should be made before its injection.

The use of large doses to prolong anaesthesia is undesirable. Many of the reports of 'hypersensitivity' reactions to propanidid involve large doses and some at least could be due to overdosage. This reminds us of the difference in the dose-response curves of thiopentone and propanidid. Large doses of the latter will often produce unsatisfactory operating conditions due to the extraneous muscular activity. The dose-related incidence of hypotension is also more noticeable with this agent. Large doses of propanidid are also likely to cause enzyme changes which are compatible with liver dysfunction.

Perhaps if propanidid were to be re-evaluated as a new induction agent and the dose restricted to that required for its safe use, then it might have a much wider acceptance than at present.

Not all the hypersensitivity reactions reported with propanidid are due to overdosage or too rapid injection. Although these are more likely to contribute to collapse after propanidid than after any other intravenous induction agent, there still remain a number of cases which are undoubtedly due to a true hypersensitivity to the drug. Propanidid releases histamine (Lorenz *et al.*, 1972), but in the normal person this probably has no special clinical significance. However, when anaphylactoid reactions have occurred, the histamine release must have been massive to produce the severe clinical signs and symptoms that ensued. The topic of hypersensitivity reactions to intravenous anaesthetics is discussed fully in Chapter 8.

In summary, propanidid is a rapidly acting non-barbiturate induction agent which is truly ultra-short-acting. It causes a high incidence of dose-related side effects, most of which can be avoided by strictly limiting the dose used. The rapid recovery time warrants a wider use of the drug in circumstances where this is of more importance than the quality of the anaesthesia produced.

References

Clarke, R. S. J. (1974). The eugenols. In: *Intravenous Anaesthesia*, pp. 162—92. Ed. by J. W. Dundee and G. M. Wyant. Churchill Livingstone, Edinburgh and London.

Clarke, R. S. J., Dundee, J. W. and Hamilton, R. C. (1967). Interactions between induction agents and muscle relaxants. *Anaesthesia* **22,** 235—48.

Doenicke, A. and Kugler, J. (1965). Electrical brain function during emergence time after methohexital and propanidid anaesthesia. *Acta anaesthesiologica Scandinavica* Suppl. 17, 99—102.

Doenicke, A., Kugler, J. and Laub, M. (1967). Evaluation of recovery and 'street fitness' by EEG and psychodiagnostic tests after anaesthesia. *Canadian Anaesthetists' Society Journal* **14,** 567—83.

Doenicke, A., Kugler, J., Schellenberger, A. and Gurtner, T. (1966). The use of electroencephalography to measure recovery time after intravenous anaesthesia. *British Journal of Anaesthesia* **38,** 580—90.

Doenicke, A., Krumey, I., Kugler, J. & Klempa, J. (1968). Experimental studies of the breakdown of Epontol: determination of propanidid in human serum. *British Journal of Anaesthesia* **40,** 415—29.

Goldman, V. and Kennedy, P. (1964). A non-barbiturate intravenous anaesthetic: report of a pilot trial. *Anaesthesia* **19,** 424—37.

Kreuscher, H. (1965). Zur Strassenverkehrstuchtigkeit nach Anwendung von Propanidid. In: *Die intravenose Kurznarkose mit dem neuen Phenoxyessigsaurederivat Propanidid (Epontol),* p. 298. Ed. by K. Horatz, R. Frey and M. Zindler. Springer-Verlag, Berlin.

Lorenz, W., Doenicke, A., Meyer, R., Reimann, J., Kusche, J., Barth, H., Geesing, H., Hutzel, M. and Weissenbacher, B. (1972). Histamine release in man by propanidid and thiopentone: pharmacological effects and clinical consequences. *British Journal of Anaesthesia* **44,** 355—69.

4

A rational approach to Althesin

This drug, which will be referred to by its proprietary name of Althesin (originally CT 1341; Alfathesin in continental Europe), is the first rapidly acting steroids to be used in routine clinical practice. A previous steroid, hydroxydione (Viadril, Presuren), enjoyed a limited popularity in the mid-1950s. There was a prolonged onset time with this preparation. It frequently took 5—10 minutes to achieve anaesthesia, and a slightly longer time before the maximum respiratory and cardiovascular depression occurred. It was, however, soluble in water — unlike the newer drug, which is insoluble. Research has continued for some time in an attempt to find a rapidly acting steroid anaesthetic which would be soluble in water but at first it appeared that such a combination was impossible (Davis and Pearce, 1972). However, there are now hopes that these difficulties have been overcome and that rapidly acting water-soluble steroid anaesthetics will soon be available for clinical trial. In the meantime we have the mixture of two steroids (alphaxalone and alphadolone acetate) in polyoxethylated castor oil — the former is the main anaesthetic agent in a concentration of 9 $mg \cdot ml^{-1}$ while the alphadolone (3 $mg \cdot ml^{-1}$ makes a small contribution to sedation but increases the solubility of alphaxalone in cremophor.

If Althesin were soluble in water, producing a less viscid solution, and if there had not been the recent spate of allergic or sensitivity reactions, then, in the opinion of the author, it would nearly approach the ideal intravenous anaesthetic.

Although Althesin was introduced initially as a satisfactory alternative to thiopentone, reasons are presented here for suggesting that this approach is no longer tenable.

Safety

In the early animal studies with Althesin, Child and his colleagues (1971) found a remarkably high therapeutic index. This is the ratio of the dose which killed half of the animals (LD_{50}) to the dose required to anaesthetize half of them (AD_{50}). Table 4.1 shows that this applied to both steroids. In this respect, Althesin was safer than the earlier hydroxydione. There was little to choose between the action of the other four drugs studied. The experimental data have real clinical application as far as the toxicity of Althesin is concerned in man. It has a very satisfactory dose-response curve with respect to cardiovascular and respiratory depression and results in the

Table 4.1 Anaesthetic and lethal doses of Althesin and some other anaesthetics by the intravenous route in male mice (Sutton, 1975)

Anaesthetic agent	AD_{50} ($mg \cdot kg^{-1}$)	LD_{50} ($mg \cdot kg^{-1}$)	Therapeutic index (LD_{50}/AD_{50})
Althesin	1.79	54.7	30.6
Hydroxydione	18.0	311.0	17.3
Thiopentone	13.2	90.5	6.9
Methohexitone	5.35	39.4	7.4
Propanidid	22.9	184.7	8.1
Ketamine	12.7	108.3	8.5

lack of untoward effects when large doses are given. Perhaps more important is the excellent tolerance of poor-risk patients to Althesin. (This is to be expected as the dose-response curve will be shifted to the right; i.e. a dose of 50 $\mu l \cdot kg^{-1}$ may exert the same depressant effect in a poor-risk subject as 100 $\mu l \cdot kg^{-1}$ in normal patients.)

Desirable properties

The speed of onset of action of Althesin is comparable with that of thiopentone but, because of viscosity and slow speed of injection, there is an impression of a longer onset time.

Like propanidid, it is miscible with water or saline solutions; this makes for easier injection and allows the use of a smaller needle. The disadvantage of these mixtures is that 'shelf life' is reduced, so any dilution should be done immediately prior to injection. The solution is slightly frothy but this does not constitute a problem. The volume of Althesin required for induction of anaesthesia (50—60 $\mu l \cdot kg^{-1}$) can be conveniently used in a 5 ml syringe, except for heavy, resistant patients. Venous thrombosis is uncommon after Althesin.

In contrast to propanidid, the duration of action of the average induction dose of Althesin is such as to allow time for a subsequent inhalation sequence. In this respect it is similar to thiopentone. Like barbiturates, it does not cause a prolongation of action of suxamethonium and it is clinically compatible with all the available non-depolarizing neuromuscular blocking drugs.

In short operations, recovery is more rapid than with thiopentone, yet not as quick as after methohexitone. One of the appealing features of this drug is the short time to full recovery of reflexes and mental clarity, compared with the usual prolonged barbiturate hangover. This is not quite as rapid as with propanidid but patients having minor operations in the morning are usually able to enjoy afternoon tea, particularly as postoperative sickness is uncommon after Althesin.

The 'quality' of anaesthesia, in terms of extraneous movement, is probably not quite as good as with thiopentone. Like other induction agents, rapid injection and the use of large doses increase the incidence of excitatory effects, and an opiate premedication reduces them. These movements are often fine and tremulous in nature and rarely interfere with the surgical procedure. Hiccough and laryngospasm are rare after Althesin.

Although one could not describe Althesin as an analgesic, it does not produce the hypersensitivity to somatic pain (antanalgesia) which is a feature of light barbiturate anaesthesia. On intermittent injection it is less cumulative than thiopentone. These two properties suggest that it might be a suitable drug for continuous administration in dilute solutions.

Effect on brain volume

One of the fascinating actions of Althesin is its effect on cerebral perfusion, cerebral metabolism and intracranial pressure. In animal experiments, Pickerodt and his colleagues (1972) found that it reduced cerebral oxygen consumption ($CMRO_2$), and that this metabolic depression led to a secondary fall in cerebral blood flow (c.b.f.) and cerebrospinal fluid pressure. These reductions may have been due in part to arterial hypotension but this is unlikely to have been the sole explanation.

In subsequent studies the Leeds workers (Turner *et al.*, 1973) found that the intravenous administration of 50 $\mu l \cdot kg^{-1}$ Althesin, to patients undergoing neurosurgery during general anaesthesia with controlled ventilation, resulted in a fall in intracranial pressure to an extent directly proportional to the starting pressure. The pressure gradually returned to the control value over 10 minutes. It was postulated that this fall in intracranial pressure was the result of a reduction in cerebral blood flow and cerebral blood volume. Takahashi and his colleagues (1973) also found a significant fall in cerebrospinal fluid pressure, their studies being carried out in normal volunteer patients. More recently, Sari *et al.* (1976) studied the cerebral circulation and metabolism in healthy patients given a single dose of 100 $\mu l \cdot kg^{-1}$, and thereafter infused at a constant rate with 0.3 $mg \cdot kg \cdot h^{-1}$ Althesin. This again demonstrated clearly that Althesin markedly reduced both the cerebral blood flow and cerebral metabolic rate, as compared with the awake state. It was accompanied by a slight increase in cerebrovascular resistance. The cerebral circulatory index (ratio of c.b.f. to $CMRO_2$) was slightly higher than that of the awake subjects but the increase was not statistically significant.

There appears to be a real use for a preparation with these actions in neurological procedures. It could be employed as a continuous infusion in a manner similar to that recommended by Savege and his colleagues (1975) for sedation in an intensive care situation. Zorab and Baskett (1977) recommend its use as the induction agent of choice in patients with head injuries, because of the rapid reversal of its action and the lack of side effects. Its potential in the field of neurological surgery does not seem to have been exploited to the full.

Hypersensitivity reactions

One cannot minimize the importance of the occurrence of hypersensitivity reactions following Althesin. Although this topic is reviewed fully in Chapter 8, it is necessary to refer to it here.

In March 1973 there were three British publications referring to immediate adverse reactions to Althesin. Jean Horton, then consultant anaesthetist at the University Hospital of Wales in Cardiff, published a straightforward report of the occurrence of an erythematous rash, with hypotension and mild oedema in a 48-year-old woman following 4.5 ml Althesin. There was no history of allergy or untoward reaction to intravenous anaesthetics, and two weeks before this event she had been given 5 ml Althesin with no untoward effects. Prompt resuscitation with cortisol and lactate—Ringer's solution was effective and the recovery was uneventful.

Concurrently, Avery and Evans (from Southampton) reported five cases of 'reactions to Althesin'. The picture is complicated in three of these by the simultaneous administration of a neuromuscular blocking drug. An 11-year-old girl, with no history of allergy, developed a crimson flush, followed by peripheral and central cyanosis (which was unresponsive to oxygen) and hypotension with tachycardia following a second administration of Althesin followed by suxamethonium. Another woman, aged 23, again with no known allergic tendency, developed severe bronchospasm on the first administration of Althesin followed by suxamethonium. A 50-year-old man, with a history of emphysema, developed bronchospasm following Althesin which was administered prior to alcuronium; this was of such severity that it nearly caused cardiac arrest. A 49-year-old woman with a history of allergies, asthma and bronchitis developed severe bronchospasm following 1 ml Althesin. Despite the use of aminophylline, cortisol and salbutamol, it was 15 minutes before adequate respiration could be established. There was a fatal outcome to the reaction which followed the administration of 2 ml Althesin in a 75-year-old asthmatic who had had no previous anaesthetics. Bronchospasm was the presenting feature and this persisted despite tracheal intubation (under paralysis induced by 50 mg suxamethonium), cortisol and aminophylline; it was eventually followed by bradycardia and cardiac arrest. Autopsy showed constriction of small bronchi and the pathologist thought that bronchospasm was present at the time of death.

The outcome was more favourable in the case reported by Joan Hester. A 35-year-old unpremedicated obese non-allergic male, who gave no history of any allergic reactions, was given 7 ml Althesin; the loss of consciousness was accompanied by coughing, clenching of teeth, bronchospasm, tachycardia (180 b.p.m.) and a diffuse erythematous rash over his face and trunk. The major signs subsided within three minutes after oxygen and cortisol were administered.

These seven case histories are quoted at length because, not only were they followed by a veritable flood of case reports, but in many ways they are typical of subsequently reported cases. Prior to the recognition of these allergic responses to intravenous anaesthetics, there had been a few reports of allergic reactions to thiopentone and a larger number following propanidid, but these few reports were overwhelmed by the interest shown in Althesin.

One important feature was that prompt treatment — mostly with steroids, fluids and oxygen — improved the recovery rate in these patients. Undoubtedly the pattern of treatment was followed by readers who encountered similar happenings. Credit must be given to Clark and Cockburn (1971) for so clearly pointing out that there was a clinical condition of 'thiopentone anaphylaxis', which was subsequently recognized as occurring with Althesin, and for clarifying its differential diagnosis and treatment.

From a perusal of these seven case reports it can be seen that three factors may play a part in predisposing to Althesin reactions: some of these patients had a history of asthma or other atopic manifestations, some had a known sensitivity to other drugs and one had a reaction only after the second administration of Althesin. Furthermore, three of these patients had a myoneural blocking drug given in conjunction with the Althesin and this could have contributed to the collapse.

These, and the subsequent spate of published cases, encouraged the author and his colleagues to request reporting on a standard form to facilitate analysis. Reactions to any form of intravenous anaesthetic were requested and an analysis of the first 100 complete reports was published by Clarke and his colleagues (1975). Ten reactions were considered to be due to causes other than the anaesthetic drug and 4 were believed to be due to a myoneural blocking drug. Of the remaining 86, 5 were described as clonic convulsions. These all occurred with Althesin and could be an exaggeration of the excitatory effects of the drug. Four occurred with propanidid, the clinical use of which was declining at that time. This left 77 reports of untoward reactions occurring with thiopentone (12) or Althesin (65). These were classified as follows (Table 4.2).

Histaminoid: reactions which could possibly be accounted for by the release of histamine. Typically there was peripheral vasodilatation, which was usually widespread, accompanied by a profound reduction in arterial pressure. The skin flush was more marked than that commonly seen at induction of anaesthesia, and oedema and weals were common.

Bronchospasm: This was often very severe and was frequently accompanied by vasodilatation or hypotension. It was sometimes preceded by coughing. In all the reported cases the bronchospasm occurred before tracheal intubation.

Cardiovascular collapse: Profound hypotension was the major problem in several patients and was not accompanied by flushing or other aspects of histaminoid reactions, although facial pallor was sometimes seen. It was not accompanied by respiratory distress.

The above reactions all occurred within one minute or so of injection of the Althesin. They often followed very small doses; a few patients complained of abdominal pain before losing consciousness.

There was another group of delayed reactions, which was limited to Althesin. The symptoms were similar in type to those classed as histaminoid but were less marked in severity, and for want of a better term these are called 'delayed histaminoid'. Their onset time was between 12 and 80 minutes after injection.

Cardiovascular collapse could be a simple manifestation of drug toxicity but a survey of the reported patients shows that this is unlikely. All received normal or even small doses, the injection was not given rapidly and there was no concomitant history of cardiac disease or the presence of hypovolaemia which would predispose to hypotension. Prior drug therapy was not a feature in these patients.

Table 4.2 Relative incidence and type of sensitivity reaction to Althesin and thiopentone, based on a report of 100 adverse reactions by Clarke *et al.*, 1975

Type of reaction	Althesin	Thiopentone	Total
Histaminoid (H)	17	2	19
Bronchospasm (B)	10	2	12
HB	25	8	33
Cardiovascular collapse	7	0	7
Delayed histaminoid	6	0	6
	65	12	77

In Table 4.2 are listed reactions which would appear to comprise a true sensitivity to the intravenous anaesthetic agent. Even assuming that the last two groups were not a true sensitivity there is still a 4:1 predominance in incidence with the steroid anaesthetic compared with thiopentone. This assumes that both drugs are used with the same frequency. As there are many more administrations of thiopentone than Althesin, one has to assume that patients are, at least, 10—20 times more prone to be hypersensitive to Althesin than to thiopentone.

With prompt treatment, there have been few fatalities among the patients having an adverse response to Althesin. There were no deaths attributed to this drug in the 65 patients reported by Clarke *et al.* (1975) as compared with 3 deaths (25 per cent) in the thiopentone series. Thus, although the frequency of reactions to Althesin is higher than that occurring with thiopentone, they are less severe than barbiturate hypersensitivity and a fatal outcome is less likely.

The increasing prevalence of hypersensitivity reactions in the population as a whole seems to be a true finding and not due simply to better reporting. Even with thiopentone there is an increasing incidence (Dundee, 1976). Nor is this phenomenon restricted to British patients, since Moneret-Vautrin, Duc and Sigiel (1976) and Vignon, Gay and Laxenaire (1976) have reported cases from France, and Fisher (1976) has reported cases from New Zealand. Mathieu and Grilliat (1976) suggest that the dose and speed of injection are causative factors in hypersensitivity reactions but this is unlikely to apply to Althesin since reactions have occurred with as little as 0.25 ml. The aetiology of the reactions is discussed fully in Chapter 8, together with their relation to histamine release and other factors.

The incidence of reactions to Althesin has been estimated to vary from about 1 in 1000 administrations (Watt, 1975; Fisher, 1976) to 1 in 18 000 (Sutton, Garrett and McArdle, 1974). In a recent survey from Wales, Evans and Keogh (1977) related the incidence found on a retrospective enquiry from anaesthetists to the total number of anesthetics given (108 708) in one hospital area over a four-year period. Their figures showed a surprisingly high incidence of adverse effects — 1 in 950 (1 in 650 to 1 in 1650) with Althesin and 1 in 14 000 (1 in 6600 to 1 in 39 300) with thiopentone. Anaesthetists may have recalled adverse reactions which they did not consider of sufficient importance to report to a national survey. If many of these responses had been life-threatening reactions, then the anaesthetists involved were failing in their obligations in not reporting these to the statutory Committee on Safety of Medicines, which in turn would have been at fault in not issuing a warning to the profession in the light of such serious evidence of drug toxicity. Two points emerge from this survey:

1. Allergic or hypersensitivity reactions to Althesin are a real problem and may reduce the usage of the drug.
2. They occur more frequently with Althesin than with thiopentone.

Other clinical indications

In the light of this, should we not now think of using Althesin in those situations where it can offer real advantages over other induction agents? Its use in neurological surgery has already been cited as an example, and by looking for other positive clinical indications we will be able to make use of the many desirable properties of this unique intravenous anaesthetic.

Outpatient anaesthesia would appear to be one of the most promising fields where Althesin offers a real alternative to methohexitone. The quality of anaesthesia is usually better with the steroid anaesthetic provided one does not inject too large doses too quickly. There is less tachycardia than following methohexitone and this is advantageous in poor-risk patients. Recovery following Althesin may not be as prompt as with methohexitone but it is quicker than after thiopentone.

The use of subanaesthetic doses of Althesin as a sedative for conservative dentistry has been described by Dixon and his colleagues (1976). They compared it with the effects of a single dose of diazepam. Both were combined with a local anaesthetic. The initial dose of Althesin was not more than 2.5 ml, with increments of 0.5 ml as required and the total dose averaged 5.4 mg (0.08 $ml \cdot kg^{-1}$). The total dose of diazepam averaged 15.3 mg (0.23 $mg \cdot kg^{-1}$). In some instances a 'cross-over' comparison between the effects of the two drugs was possible. In general, the operating conditions were not as good with Althesin, due to the occurrence of tremor and shivering. In contrast to diazepam, verbal contact was lost with the patient following that first dose of Althesin. The cardiovascular and respiratory effects were similar for both drugs.

As a test of recovery, patients were asked to cross out, in three minutes, a designated letter on a specially designed sheet containing lines of jumbled letters. Recovery was considered to be complete when this had returned to predrug levels. There were such wide differences between the recovery times with the two techniques that these are summarized in Table 4.3. More patients had recovered 10 minutes after leaving the chair following Althesin than after 30 minutes following diazepam. Arm soreness was more common (34 per cent) after diazepam than following Althesin (15 per cent). The anxiolytic action of subanaesthetic doses of Althesin was at least as good as that of diazepam.

Table 4.3 Percentage incidence of patients who are considered to have 'recovered' from the effects of diazepam or Althesin, used for sedation in conservative dentistry

	All patients		Cross-over studies	
	Diazepam	Althesin	Diazepam	Althesin
Number	45	52	36	36
Time from leaving chair:				
10 min	2	37	3	36
20 min	20	48	22	53
30 min	29	69	31	72

From Dixon *et al.* (1976)

Without entering into controversy on the use of light anaesthesia techniques for conservative dentistry, one can see advantages from the use of Althesin in this field. In a non-hospital situation rapid recovery may be more important than perfect operating conditions. However, since there was always a period of actual anaesthesia with Althesin, it is essential to have an anaesthetist or a person other than the operator who can look after the airway and, if necessary, carry out resuscitation should an acute hypersensitivity occur. Diazepam, in low doses, results in sedation rather than anaesthesia and is preferable for the single-handed operator. If the choice is between Althesin and methohexitone, then the steroid may be preferred because of the lower incidence of tachycardia. Both are preferable to propanidid, which results in uneven anaesthesia and causes a high incidence of venous damage.

Obstetrics is a field in which the prompt recovery from Althesin could be used to advantage but whether it has any special advantages here is open to question. This could also apply to anaesthesia for endoscopy and for operations such as tonsillectomy where an active cough reflex is essential at the end of the operation. Being a non-barbiturate, one might suggest its use in patients with known or suspected porphyria but there is evidence that Althesin may affect ALA synthetase in a manner similar to the barbiturates; it should *not* be used in these patients.

Infusions

Concern over pollution of the operating room atmosphere with anaesthetic gases and vapors led Savege and his colleagues (1975) to explore the potential of continuous infusion of a dilute (10 per cent) solution of Althesin as a means of maintaining sleep. Workers from the same institution (The London Hospital) have previously reported its use as a sedative in an intensive therapy unit (Ramsay *et al.*, 1974). In this latter field it allowed rapid and accurate control of the level of sedation. It was considered to have two particularly useful applications: it provided 'light sleep' and permitted rapid variation in the level of sedation, allowing repeated assessment of the central nervous system to be made. The technique proved to be particularly valuable in patients who needed intermittent periods of controlled ventilation, in restless and confused patients (especially those with cerebral trauma) and in patients in whom large doses of conventional sedatives were ineffective.

No side effects of sufficient severity to justify stopping the infusion occurred and none lasted for more than 30 minutes or needed treatment. Muscle twitching, hiccough, nausea, salivation and flushing of the skin were reported. There was no evidence of upper respiratory tract obstruction and, apart from the initial tachycardia, the cardiovascular effects were insignificant. Althesin was given with analgesics and neuromuscular blocking drugs as required and no adverse interactions were noted.

As an index of its safety, the infusion was continued for periods of up to 20 days without evidence of tachyphylaxis or delay in the recovery time. The total volume of (undiluted) Althesin administered was as high as 4.37 litres in one patient (a myasthenic) and six other patients received doses in excess of 1 litre. Liver function tests, haemoglobin and other estimations were carried out every third day. Three patients developed changes suggestive of liver dysfunction but these were readily explicable on non-drug clinical grounds. Four other patients showed slight changes which were not unexpected after the clinical course of their illnesses and which were of short duration. The three patients who underwent the longest period of sedation had liver function test results within the normal range.

One may hesitate to recommend the use of continuous Althesin infusion as an alternative to conventional forms of anaesthesia but it may be worth while pursuing in the intensive care situation. The technique for anaesthesia is described fully by Savege *et al.* (1975) and is similar to that for sedation. A few practical points are worth noting. The infusion system incorporates a 100 ml burette which is used to measure accurately the quantity of drug given and also acts as a safety device to prevent accidental administration of a large quantity of drug. A three-way tap allows a bolus dose to be given (for induction) and also the administration of other drugs. A predetermined dose can be given with a constant-rate infusion pump of the Ivac type.

To overcome the lack of analgesia with Althesin, the infusions have been combined with parenteral analgesics, particularly with pentazocine. Dechene (1977) infused dilute Althesin (10 ml added to 120 ml dextrose-water), giving 120 $\mu l \cdot kg^{-1}$ over 3—4 minutes for induction and maintaining sleep with 2.7 μl·kg·min^{-1}. To this he added pentazocine, starting with 6—12 mg and incremental doses of 6 mg as required. The administration of the analgesic was discontinued before the end of the anaesthetic. He also gave nitrous oxide—oxygen, thus defeating any attempt to prevent theatre pollution by this technique. The method he describes really only substitutes Althesin infusion for a volatile supplement. Relaxation was produced by specific drugs where appropriate. In his report on 409 cases he comments that this technique is justified on ecological grounds, a comment which seems scarcely appropriate.

Jago and Restall (1977) employed the same drugs, but gave these intermittently, rather than by infusion. They also avoided nitrous oxide. Many of their 208 patients were rather heavily premedicated and this may account for the good quality of anaesthesia. One hopes that others will continue to explore the possibilities of continuous infusion or intermittent administration of Althesin and analgesics, and that it will soon be possible to assess the potential of this technique.

Malignant hyperpyrexia

Honda and colleagues (1977) from Japan have recently reported the uneventful use of Althesin in two patients who were already identified as being susceptible to malignant hyperpyrexia. Both of these patients received halothane. Considered together with previous reports by Page, Morgan and Loh (1972) and Judelman and Pirie (1974), this suggests that Althesin has some protective action and may be the agent of choice in susceptible patients.

Personal assessment

In Althesin, we have a unique intravenous anaesthetic. Its insolubility in water is a disadvantage but the viscosity caused by the solvent can be overcome by dilution. It is useful as an induction agent, as part of a balanced anaesthetic technique, and its relative lack of toxicity is a real advantage in poor-risk patients. Had it been free from hypersensitivity reactions, it may well have offered a real challenge to thiopentone.

Until about five years ago there were a few sporadic reports of cases of so-called 'hypersensitivity' to intravenous anaesthetics and this subject has only achieved clinical importance since Althesin was introduced. To suggest that the problem is unconnected with the introduction of the steroid anaesthetic is unrealistic, although there is good evidence that drug sensitivity to all types of drugs is becoming more common. More and more people in the community are taking tranquillizers or analgesics, and the widespread use of oral contraceptives may play a part. Thus we had a drug which was more prone to cause hypersensitivity reactions and, furthermore, it was introduced at a time when the patient population was more likely to react adversely to drugs. The dramatic hypotensive episodes, often associated with bronchospasm and hypoxia, are life-threatening. Had they occurred in a medical discipline not so adept at handling acute emergencies, the results would have been disastrous. At best, these episodes are frightening, but recovery usually occurs very quickly and only a few fatalities have been reported.

Nevertheless, the situation is sufficiently serious as to suggest limiting the use of Althesin to specific situations where it offers advantages. Research is needed in this field to explore the possibility of using Althesin in neurological operations, in patients with head injuries or even after cardiac arrest or hypoxic episodes. There should be an indication for the use of a drug which causes such a reduction in cerebral metabolic activity.

Other indications are less clear; hypersensitivity is not dose-related and thus the light anaesthesia or sedation recommended in dental practice or the use of infusions of dilute solutions are, theoretically, not free from the risks of these reactions. This is a fruitful field for clinical research, which should be carried out only by experienced investigators in a well equipped hospital.

We have no means of knowing whether newer steroid anaesthetics would be free from the risk of adverse reactions. Three years elapsed between the first clinical paper on Althesin and the report of a hypersensitivity reaction. Perhaps the research projects referred to in Chapter 8 may eventually clarify the relationship between the chemical structure of steroids and their likelihood to cause hypersensitivity. Elimination of the need for a solubilizing agent will at least remove one possible a factor. A rapidly acting water-soluble steroid anaesthetic would seem likely to offer great potential.

References

Avery, A. F. and Evans, A. (1973). Reactions to Althesin. *British Journal of Anaesthesia* **45**, 301—3.

Child, K. J., Currie, J. P., Davis, B., Dodds, M. G., Pearce, D. R. and Twissell, D. J. (1971). The pharmacological properties in animals of CT 1341 — a new steroid anaesthetic agent. *British Journal of Anaesthesia* **43**, 2—13.

Clark, M. M. and Cockburn, H. A. (1971). Anaphylactoid response to thiopentone. *British Journal of Anaesthesia* **43**, 185—9.

Clarke, R. S. J., Dundee, J. W., Garrett, R. T., McArdle, G. K. and Sutton, J. A. (1975). Adverse reactions to intravenous anaesthetics. A survey of 100 reports. *British Journal of Anaesthesia* **47**, 575-85.

Davis, B. and Pearce, D. R. (1972). An introduction to Althesin (CT 1341). *Postgraduate Medical Journal* **48**, Suppl. 2, 13—17.

Dechene, J. P. (1977). Alfathesin by continuous infusion supplemented with intermittent pentazocine. *Canadian Anaesthetists' Society Journal* **24**, 702—6.

Dixon, R. A., Atkinson, R. W., Kenyon, C., Lamb, D., Thornton, J. A. and Woodhead, S. (1976). Subanaesthetic dosage of Althesin as a sedative for conservative dentistry. *British Journal of Anaesthesia* **48**, 431—9.

Dundee, J. W. (1976). Hypersensitivity to intravenous anaesthetics. *British Journal of Anaesthesia* **48,** 57—8.

Evans, J. M. and Keogh, J. A. M. (1977). Adverse reactions to intravenous anaesthetic induction agents. *British Medical Journal* **2,** 735-6.

Fisher, M. M. (1976). Severe histamine mediated reactions to Althesin. *Anaesthesia and Intensive Care* **4,** 33—5.

Hester, J. B. (1973). Reaction to Althesin. *British Journal of Anaesthesia* **45,** 303.

Honda, N., Konno, K., Itohda, Y., Nishino, M., Matsushima, S., Haseba, S., Honda, Y. and Gotoh, Y. (1977). Malignant hyperthermia and Althesin. *Canadian Anaesthetists' Society Journal* **24,** 514—21.

Horton, J. N. (1973). Adverse reaction to Althesin. *Anaesthesia* **28,** 182—3.

Jago, R. H. & Restall, J. (1977). Total intravenous anaesthesia. A technique based on alphaxalone/alphadolone and pentazocine. *Anaesthesia* **32,** 904—7.

Judelman, H. and Pirie, D. H. (1974). Anaesthesia in a patient with previous malignant hyperpyrexia. *British Journal of Anaesthesia* **46,** 519.

Mathieu, A. and Grilliat, J. P. (1976). Correspondence. *British Journal of Anaesthesia* **48,** 49—50.

Moneret-Vautrin, D. A., Duc, M. and Sigiel, M. (1976). Etude de différents facteurs de risque du déclenchement d'accidents aux anesthésiques et myorelaxants. *Annales de l'Anesthésiologie Française* **17,** 165—74.

Page, P., Morgan, M. and Loh, L. (1972). Ketamine anaesthesia in paediatric procedures. *Acta anaesthesiologica Scandinavica* **16,** 155—60.

Pickerodt, V., McDowall, D. G., Coroneos, N. J. and Keaney, N. P. (1972). Effect of Althesin on carotid blood flow and intracranial pressure in the anaesthetised baboon: a preliminary communication. *Postgraduate Medical Journal* **48,** Suppl. 2, 58—61.

Ramsay, M. A. E., Savege, T. M., Simpson, B. R. J. and Goodwin, R. (1974). Controlled sedation with alphaxalone—alphadolone. *British Medical Journal* **2,** 656—9.

Sari, A., Maekawa, T., Tohjo, M., Okuda, Y. and Takeshita, H. (1976). Effects of Althesin on cerebral blood flow and oxygen consumption in man. *British Journal of Anaesthesia* **48,** 545—50.

Savege, T. M., Ramsay, M. A. E., Curran, J. P. J., Cotter, J., Walling, P. T. and Simpson, B. R. (1975). Intravenous anaesthesia by infusion: a technique using alphaxalone/alphadolone (Althesin). *Anaesthesia* **30,** 757—64.

Sutton, J. A. (1975). Alfatesin: Animal Pharmacology in relation to clinical anaesthesia. In *Recent Progress in Anaesthesiology and Resuscitation.* Proceedings of the IV European Congress of Anaesthesiology, Madrid 5—11 September 1974. Edited by A. Arias, R. Llaurado, M. A. Nalda and J. N. Lunn, p. 87—93. Excerpta Medica, Amsterdam.

Sutton, J. A., Garrett, R. T. and McArdle, G. K. (1974). A survey of adverse reactions to Althesin. *British Journal of Anaesthesia* **46,** 806.

Takahashi, T., Takasaki, M., Namiki, A. and Dohi, A. (1973). Effects of Althesin on cerebrospinal fluid pressure. *British Journal of Anaesthesia* **45,** 179—84.

Turner, J. M., Coroneos, N. J., Gibson, R. M., Powell, D., Ness, M. A. and McDowall, D. G. (1973). The effect of Althesin on intracranial pressure in man. *British Journal of Anaesthesia* **45,** 168—72.

Vignon, H., Gay, R. and Laxenaire, M. C. (1976). Observations cliniques d'accidents anaphylactoides per et post anesthésiques. Resultat d'enquêtes a posteriore. *Annales de l'Anésthesiologie Française* **17,** 117—21.

Watt, J. M. (1975). Anaphylactic reactions after use of CT 1341 (Althesin). *British Medical Journal* **3,** 205—6.

Zorab, J. S. M. and Baskett, P. J. F. (1977). *Immediate Care.* W. B. Saunders, London.

5

Pros and cons of ketamine

There is little dispute as to the advantages of this unique agent. It is soluble in water and can be given by both the intramuscular and intravenous routes. In contrast to the barbiturates, ketamine solutions have a less alkaline pH, in the range of 3.5—5.5, and they are non-irritant on injection. It is available commercially in solution containing 10, 50 and 100 $mg \cdot ml^{-1}$, the last being reserved almost exclusively for intramuscular injection. Ketamine does not appear to have any antanalgesic action; in fact, analgesia is one of its prominent and desirable properties. Opinions differ as to whether this analgesia is sufficient for all abdominal surgery, especially that requiring opening the peritoneum. Although Corssen and Domino (1966) suggest that it may be inadequate for this purpose and that its use should be limited to producing what they call 'somatoanalgesia', other anaesthetists (Gibbs, 1977; Sabathie *et al.*, 1977), including the authors of this chapter, have found it to be very satisfactory as the main agent for patients undergoing major abdominal operations.

Unlike thiopentone, there is delay of between 30 and 90 seconds to the onset of sleep when ketamine is given intravenously and between 2 and 8 minutes when it is given by intramuscular injection. If the intramuscular route is used, care must be taken to ensure that the drug is injected deep into muscle for there can be an even longer latent period if it is injected into subcutaneous fat.

Ketamine may have a twofold action on cerebral activity, depressing the non-specific diffusely projecting thalamic system in selected areas of neocortex (especially the association areas and sensory and motor cortex) while simultaneously stimulating parts of the limbic system. It appears to have minimal action on the reticular activating system and the thalamic sensory nuclei, and in this respect it is different from most other anaesthetic agents (Moruzzi and Magoun, 1949; French, Verzeano and Magoun, 1953). This dual effect led Domino, Chodoff and Corssen (1965) to coin the phrase 'dissociative anaesthesia' to describe the state produced by ketamine. This has two important clinical implications. First, children under 6 months require proportionately larger doses than adults and it may not be possible to induce surgical anaesthesia in patients with severe brain injuries. Secondly, the 'type' of anaesthesia is different from that of orthodox techniques in that the patients exhibit some degree of catalepsy and may remain apparently deeply anaesthetized with their eyes open.

It is not proposed to discuss the advantages or the clinical usefulness of ketamine in any depth but rather to relate its advantages to its disadvantages and to look at attempts which are currently being made to overcome the latter. Figure 5.1 summarizes the present position as seen by the authors. In the absence of attempts to attenuate the side effects — particularly those occurring during the recovery period — then the advantages of ketamine do not outweigh the disadvantages and one is left with a very limited field of use for the drug, in paediatric anaesthesia and perhaps in situations such as repeated burn dressings. However, with the use of appropriate medication, which will minimize some of these sequelae, then the disadvantages are less marked. Nevertheless, at present it must be admitted that the side effects of ketamine are such as to limit its widespread use. If one considers the small number of anaesthetists who use the drug at all, it becomes clear that the many advantages of the drug are not sufficient to overcome the problems associated with its use, particularly in the early postoperative period.

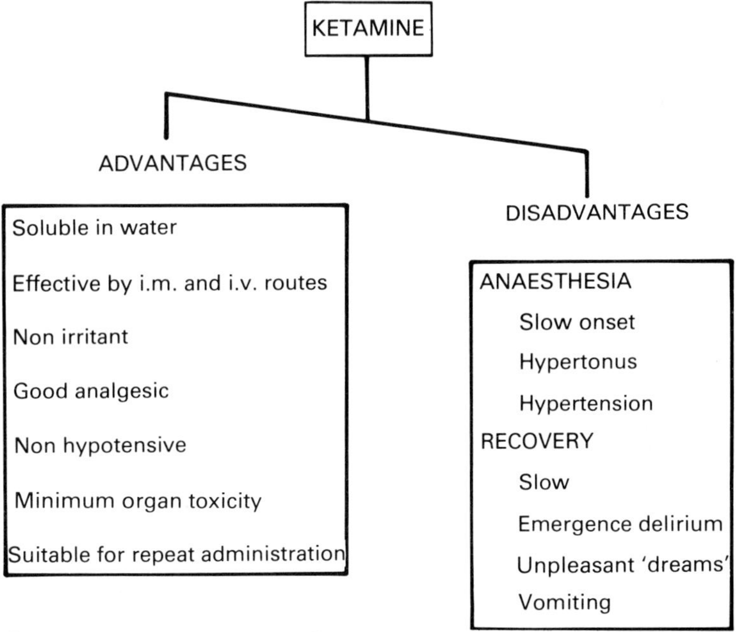

Fig. 5.1 The present status of ketamine?

Induction of anaesthesia

The slow onset of anaesthesia is not a major disadvantage provided it is anticipated. Hypertonus, however, can be a problem and it is accentuated by giving high doses. On occasions it may be difficult to distinguish between hypertonus and light anaesthesia, and this can result in an overdose of ketamine. The author has come across situations where hypertonus has interfered with positioning a patient on the operating table and it has been necessary to resort to other drugs. Respiratory complications do not occur frequently during induction of anaesthesia with ketamine.

Although the laryngeal reflexes are not markedly depressed with clinical doses of ketamine, the extent to which protective reflexes remain intact is not as great as was originally suggested (Taylor and Towey, 1971; Carson *et al.*, 1973). The latter study showed that the addition of any depressant premedication would reduce the activity of these protective reflexes; however, it may be necessary to give preoperative medication to avoid unpleasant sequelae. Diazepam, opiates and droperidol all depress laryngeal reflexes. Generally speaking, jaw tone is well maintained during light ketamine anaesthesia and this is certainly advantageous, but limits its use for laryngoscopy.

The remainder of this chapter is concentrated on some aspects of the side effects of ketamine and of its use by continuous infusion.

Cardiovascular system

In contrast to most conventional anaesthetics, some degree of cardiovascular stimulation almost invariably occurs with ketamine. This affects both blood pressure and heart rate. In the absence of a depressant premedication, the rise in systolic pressure in adults receiving clinical doses of 1–2 $mg \cdot kg^{-1}$ is usually in the range of 20–40 mmHg, with a slightly lower rise in diastolic pressure. In the majority of patients the blood pressure rises steadily over the first 3–5 minutes following injection of a single bolus and then declines to normal limits within the next 10–20 minutes. There is often a slight delay in the rise in diastolic pressure, which may still be rising when the systolic is declining.

There is wide individual variation in the cardiovascular response to ketamine and occasionally alarming increases in pressure can occur. However, the authors have monitored closely the changes in some 4000 administrations to adults and they have encountered no problems arising from the rise in blood pressure. Ketamine nearly always causes an increase in heart rate in man.

Much has been written on the subject of ketamine-induced hypertension and many unsubstantiated statements appear in the literature. Despite views to the contrary, there is very little evidence of a dose-related response with amounts above 1 $mg \cdot kg^{-1}$; a hypertensive response to ketamine can occur with subhypnotic doses but it is less marked. Neither the rate of injection nor the route of administration has much effect on the degree of hypertension. Contrary to an early opinion, the initial level of blood pressure does not appear to affect the degree of hypertension nor does the age of the patient influence the response. There is no basis for the belief that hypertensive patients are less susceptible to this hypertensive response than normotensive or even hypotensive subjects.

Most premedicants will decrease the rise in blood pressure to some degree, as will tubocurarine. However, when ketamine is given with pancuronium, the rise in pressure is greater than when tubocurarine or alcuronium are used. Tachycardia is also greater with a ketamine—pancuronium sequence than with ketamine alone or in combination with alcuronium or tubocurarine. Ketamine causes a rise in cardiac output which is mainly due to an increase in heart rate rather than stroke volume. It has a negative inotropic action on isolated mammalian heart and even extremely large doses (20 $mg \cdot kg^{-1}$) have no stimulatory action on the myocardium. Since the effect on the denervated myocardium is one of depression, the hypertension and tachycardia which occur under clinical conditions are probably due to sympathetic overactivity. A rise in circulating noradrenaline following the administration of ketamine has been demonstrated by several workers. The ability of halothane, high epidural anaesthesia and phentolamine to prevent the pressor response is indirect evidence of the involvement of the sympathetic nervous system. It has been suggested that this sympathetic stimulation is centrally mediated but animal studies show that ketamine desensitizes the arterial baroreceptors, thereby reducing negative feedback mechanism to the vasomotor centre, with resulting hypertension and tachycardia. This peripheral site of action resembles that of diethyl ether and cyclopropane, and would be in keeping with the production of an increased level of circulating catecholamines. A cocaine-like effect — preventing re-uptake of noradrenaline by adrenergic nerve terminals — also occurs and is a likely explanation for the hypertensive action of ketamine.

Apart from the established observation that hypertension is less marked in patients who have received heavy premedication, and the work of Johnstone (1976) with verapamil, there have been no published studies on the results of any attempt to attenuate the cardiovascular effects of ketamine. Verapamil is a derivative of papaverine and blocks the uptake by the myocardial cells of ionized calcium which is necessary for the breakdown of ATP. This action reduces myocardial contractility and is referred to as a negative inotropic action. Lilburn, Moore and Dundee (1978) have tried the effects of pretreatment or administration during anaesthesia of a large number of alpha and beta adrenergic and ganglion blocking drugs on the hypertension which occurs during infusions of ketamine. These included practolol and phentolamine, either alone or in combination, and promethazine, hexamethonium and procainamide. None of these was effective in reducing heart rate and blood pressure changes. Verapamil in doses of 10—15 mg was injected intravenously over one minute immediately after the induction of anaesthesia and, although this attenuated the rise in blood pressure, the increase in heart rate was greater in patients who received the verapamil than in the control group.

The alpha and beta adrenergic blocking drug, labetalol, was also studied. Preliminary results obtained with this drug are promising. It was given in doses of 0.5 and 1.0 $mg \cdot kg^{-1}$ simultaneously with ketamine. The blood pressure was less well controlled than was heart rate.

To compare the effects of different drugs, Lilburn, Moore and Dundee (1978) graded the degree of attenuation as follows:

Blood pressure

Good = rise in systolic and diastolic of less than 20 mmHg at any time.
Poor = persistent (at least 5 minutes) rise in diastolic pressure of 40 mmHg and/or diastolic of 30 mmHg.
Fair = intermediate between above.

Heart rate

Good = rise of less than 20 beats/min.
Poor = persistent (5 minutes) rise of 40 beats/min.
Fair = intermediate between above.

Table 5.1 compares the effects of two doses of labetalol with those of verapamil using these criteria. This shows that the adrenergic blocking drug has a more beneficial effect. In subsequent studies, Dundee, Lilburn and Moore (1978) used the same doses of labetalol in patients anaesthetized with ketamine infusions and paralysed by tubocurarine. Tubocurarine often led to a fall in blood pressure in patients receiving the large dose of labetalol and is not recommended. Taken together, these findings are disappointing and one has no certain, safe way of preventing the cardiostimulatory effects of ketamine. Should there be a specific indication for ketamine, then the concomitant administration of a low concentration of halothane will keep the blood pressure within normal limits. This, however, defeats many of the advantages of ketamine, particularly its use as sole anaesthetic.

Table 5.1 Comparison of the attenuation of the cardiostimulatory effects of ketamine by verapamil and labetalol in three groups, each of 10 patients

Blood pressure control				Heart rate control		
Verapamil 10–15 mg	Labetalol ($mg \cdot kg^{-1}$)			Verapamil 10–15 mg	Labetalol ($mg \cdot kg^{-1}$)	
	0.5	1.0			0.5	1.0
4	4	3	Good	0	8	9
4	5	7	Fair	4	2	1
2	1	0	Poor	6	0	0

Ketamine—labetalol is not without its dangers, as Fig. 5.2 shows. Three doses of labetalol failed to control the blood pressure rise in this 58-year-old 55 kg woman, anaesthetized with a ketamine infusion following an initial dose of 55 mg of the drug and given supplementary doses as indicated. Three doses, each of 30 mg labetalol, failed to control the rise in pressure and 5 mg droperidol was given. This patient underwent two operations — a breast biopsy which was followed by mastectomy. The combination of labetalol and droperidol made the patient very sensitive to a moderate blood loss and the hypotension was such that a rapid infusion of 500 ml of dextran 70 was required. This quickly restored blood pressure to within normal limits.

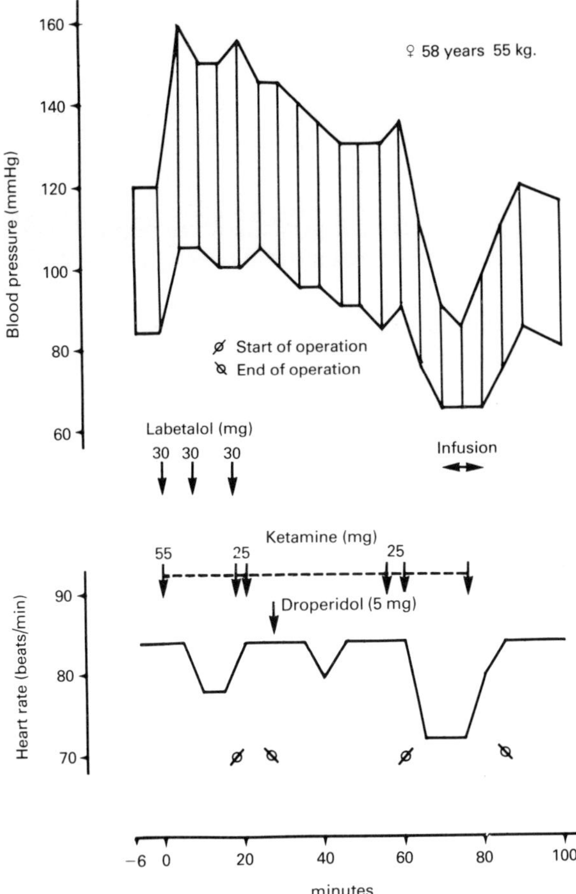

Fig. 5.2 Systolic and diastolic blood pressure in a patient anaesthetized with a ketamine infusion (---) and given supplementary doses as shown. This patient underwent two operations. A rapid infusion of 500 ml dextran 70 quickly restored blood pressure to within normal limits.

Recovery problems

Recovery is slower after ketamine than after conventional intravenous drugs but this need cause no problems as patients are usually in full control of their reflexes. Nausea and vomiting appear to occur somewhat more frequently than with other techniques but again this is not a major problem and the preoperative administration of anti-emetics is not recommended as a routine.

Serious psychotomimetic effects have occurred after all 'dissociative drugs' and these led to the abandonment of phencyclidine as an intravenous anaesthetic. The effects of ketamine are qualitatively similar to those of its predecessor but are of considerably shorter duration.

There are two important aspects of recovery which have to be considered:

1. *Emergence delirium or excitement*. This occurs in the immediate post-operative period and the patients become disorientated, extremely restless and agitated. It is often accompanied by irrational talking or uncontrolled crying or moaning.
2. *Vivid dreams or hallucinations.* These can occur up to 24 hours after ketamine; frequently they have a morbid content and are often experienced in vivid technicolour.

Emergence delirium or excitement does not upset the patients themselves as they are unaware of its occurrence. However, it does upset nurses and other attendants and is very undesirable in a situation where patients waiting to come to operation may become aware of the disturbance. In contrast, the vivid dreams or hallucinations do upset the patients, particularly when they have morbid or unpleasant content. The attendants may be unaware of these, which can be of such severity as to deter patients from having subsequent anaesthetics. Perhaps they are most important in patients who have had previous anaesthetics with orthodox drugs and who have not experienced this occurrence.

Table 5.2 lists a number of factors which are thought to influence the incidence and severity of emergence disturbances. It is generally assumed that these do not occur in children, particularly in the very young, but one can never be sure of this. Perhaps failure to record them indicates inability to communicate rather than the fact that they have not occurred. The influence of the nature of the operation and the duration of anaesthesia are interrelated. A number of people have found that they occur less frequently after body surface operations of 30—40 minutes' duration than after minor procedures lasting 5—10 minutes. They are uncommon after prolonged surgery. It has been suggested that disturbing the patient during the arousal period is likely to cause emergence delirium but this is not proven.

Table 5.2 Factors thought to influence the incidence and severity of emergence delirium from ketamine

1. Uncommon in children and elderly
2. Females more prone than males
3. Absence of premedication
4. Nature of operation
5. Duration of anaesthesia
6. Disturbance during arousal
7. Frequency of use*

*Less frequent on repeated use

It is more difficult to look at the incidence of dreaming because many patients, particularly those given nitrous oxide, have postoperative dreams and this is only remarked upon when the content of the dreams is unpleasant. As an example of this, children often get postoperative dreams and although these may occur more frequently after ketamine, they do not seem to upset the children nor do they appear to have a morbid content. King and Stephen

(1967) have found an incidence of hallucinations as high as 50 per cent in adults and Iwatsuki *et al.* (1967) have reported a 77 per cent incidence.

Visual disturbances, which may also be influenced by premedication, occur after ketamine and these can lead to both delirium and hallucinations. Their severity varies from patient to patient but the 'sensory and perceptual' misinterpretations which occur obviously are of importance.

The importance of disagreeable dreams and visual disturbances is shown by the number of patients who would not be prepared to have ketamine again should they require a similar operation. Knox *et al.* (1970), in one of the early British studies, found this figure to be 53 per cent in unpremedicated patients. More recently, Morgan *et al.* (1971) found that only 10 per cent of his patients were unwilling to have the same anaesthetic again.

Heavy premedication such as opiate—hyoscine or opiate—hyoscine—droperidol is effective in reducing emergence delirium but has less effect in preventing unpleasant dreams. Intravenous droperidol, given near the end of the operation, is also effective against emergence delirium but is ineffective against preventing the occurrence of dreams. In contrast, intravenous diazepam, although being ineffective against emergence delirium, reduces the incidence of unpleasant dreams. An oral mixture of 10 mg nitrazepam and 20 mg droperidol has been recommended for patients undergoing abdominal operations with ketamine as the main anaesthetic (Johnstone, 1972) and this is reported to reduce all the sequelae.

It is generally agreed that there is an unacceptably high incidence of emergence sequelae when ketamine is used for induction or as the main agent for minor gynaecological procedures. Using these patients as a 'study model' the authors have investigated the influence of a large number of drugs given either before or at the end of operation, in the hope of finding a suitable premedicant which would retain the desirable features of ketamine anaesthesia and yet make it more acceptable both to the patients and their attendants.

In a systematic study of the ability of various premedicants to attenuate the psychic actions of ketamine, Lilburn and his colleagues (1978) induced anaesthesia with 2 $mg \cdot kg^{-1}$ ketamine and maintained it with intermittent doses in the region of 0.25 $mg \cdot kg^{-1}$. Patients were observed closely at the end of operation and the occurrence and severity of emergence delirium were noted. At a visit made 6 or 24 hours after operation they were questioned about the occurrence of 'dreams' which were classed as unpleasant or pleasant according to their content. At this visit patients were asked if, in the event of their requiring a similar operation, they would be happy to have the same anaesthetic on a subsequent occasion.

In the first part of the study a large number of drugs was given intravenously 10 minutes before the induction of anaesthesia to groups of at least 20 patients. Drugs used included benzodiazepines, neurolept combinations or standard premedicants.

Benzodiazepines. Diazepam was given in doses of 15 mg and 0.2 $mg \cdot kg^{-1}$. The newer benzodiazepine, flunitrazepam, was given in one-tenth of these doses and the longer acting lorazepam was given in 4 mg doses. A mixture of the short-acting diazepam (5 mg) and the longer-acting lorazepam (2 mg) was also tried.

Neurolept combinations. These consisted of droperidol 5 mg, with or without fentanyl 0.1 mg, and a combination of trifluoperazine 2 mg and fentanyl 0.05 mg.

Standard premedications. Reflecting American practice, pentobarbitone 100 mg and hydroxyzine 100 mg were given; reflecting British practice, pethidine 100 mg and promethazine 25 mg were included.

Controls. In view of the known incidence of unpleasant side effects in unpremedicated patients, the control series was kept very small but it was thought justifiable to include data from similar studies carried out by the same workers in the same department (this gave a total of 45 patients).

In Table 5.3 the results with the two doses of diazepam and with the two doses of flunitrazepam are pooled as are the results from all the neurolept combinations. It was not possible to complete the studies in patients pre-medicated with pethidine 100 mg or with pentobarbitone 100 mg because of the poor quality of anaesthesia. It can be seen from these results that flunitrazepam and lorazepam are both very effective in reducing the morbid content of postoperative dreams and making anaesthesia acceptable to the patient. Promethazine is also effective in this respect but it was usually followed by an excessively high level of emergence delirium.

Table 5.3 Percentage incidence of emergence delirium, postoperative unpleasant 'dreams' and unacceptable anaesthesia in women undergoing minor gynaecological operations under intermittent ketamine anaesthesia with the premedicants shown given intravenously 10—15 minutes prior to induction

Premedication	Emergence delirium	Unpleasant 'dreams'	Anaesthesia unacceptable to patient
Control (saline)	47	33	64
Diazepam	35	15	23
Flunitrazepam	35	2	7
Lorazepam	10	2	4
Neurolept combination	16	22	22
Hydroxyzine	15	35	35
Promethazine	30	20	0

In the second part of the study the effect of the three benzodiazepines was studied in more detail. In this case the premedication was given 30—40 minutes before induction of anaesthesia, and again there was a minimum number of 20 patients in each series.

Table 5.4 shows the superiority of lorazepam over the other two drugs, and this seems to be a genuine advance in the attenuation of the ketamine sequelae.

Table 5.4 Percentage incidence of postoperative sequelae in women undergoing minor gynaecological operations under ketamine anaesthesia when this was preceded by intravenous benzodiazepines 30–40 minutes before induction

	Severe or prolonged emergence delirium	Unpleasant 'dreams'	Anaesthesia unacceptable to patient
Diazepam 15 mg or 0.2 $mg \cdot kg^{-1}$	45	20	30
Flunitrazepam 1.5 mg or 0.02 $mg \cdot kg^{-1}$	15	10	5
Lorazepam 4 mg	0	0	0

In subsequent studies lorazepam was administered intramuscularly and orally; the 4 mg dose is effective by either of these routes. However, reducing this dose to the commercially available 2.5 mg tablet still leaves an unacceptably high incidence of emergence delirium or other unpleasant sequelae from ketamine. The 4 mg dose is followed by a more delayed recovery than one would like and in minor operations one may lose many of the advantages of ketamine; nevertheless, it is effective in completely abolishing sequelae. We have given this dose both orally and intravenously before ketamine infusions in which very large doses of ketamine were used, and it was effective in reducing sequelae and in making the anaesthetic acceptable to the patient (Dundee and Lilburn, 1978; Lilburn, Dundee and Moore, 1978).

Ketamine infusions

Despite its many disadvantages, ketamine may offer a potential answer to the problem of pollution of the operating theatre by gases and vapours (Chapter 11). It is a relatively long-acting drug with a good analgesic action and does not require supplementing with nitrous oxide. Lorazepam premedication eliminates problems of emergence delirium and postoperative dreams, which made an exploration of this field not only ethically justified, but also desirable. Lilburn, Dundee and Moore (1978) have reported observations on its use in over 200 major surgical procedures. After an induction dose of 1 $mg \cdot kg^{-1}$ they continued with an infusion containing 1 $mg \cdot ml^{-1}$ in 5 per cent dextrose or balanced salt solution. Supplementary doses of 0.5 $mg \cdot kg^{-1}$ were given when the infusion did not provide an adequate depth of anaesthesia.

With inhalational anaesthesia one can always give a basal concentration of nitrous oxide or volatile supplements which will be certain to keep the patient asleep. This does not apply with ketamine infusions. Accordingly, our initial studies were performed with patients breathing spontaneously. The average dose requirement was calculated from this study before starting the series with controlled ventilation. It was soon found that one was inclined to overdose the patients who were breathing spontaneously because of hypertonus. By abolishing hypertonus the myoneural blocking drugs reduced the ketamine requirements. There was however, a lower limit for this dose reduction below which one did not feel certain that the patients would not be aware of the operation.

Nitrous oxide was not used at all. There was no incompatibility between ketamine and the myoneural blocking drugs, and no problems of reversal of the block with neostigmine were encountered.

Table 5.5 lists our recommendations on dosage. It will be noted that these are given as $mg \cdot kg^{-1}$ at 10-minute intervals rather than as $mg \cdot kg^{-1} \cdot min^{-1}$ or $mg \cdot kg^{-1} \cdot h^{-1}$ as in some publications. A minute-by-minute dosage can be misleading because, as anaesthesia proceeds, the ketamine requirements become reduced so that the dose in $mg \cdot kg^{-1} \cdot min^{-1}$ appears to be much smaller for a 60-minute operation than for a 20-minute procedure.

Table 5.5 Approximate average total dose of ketamine ($mg \cdot kg^{-1}$) required to maintain an adequate depth of anaesthesia in adults premedicated with 4 mg lorazepam

Time (min)	Controlled ventilation	Spontaneous ventilation
Initial	1.0	1.0
10	1.9–2.0	2.2
20	2.7–2.8	3.4–3.5
30	3.4–3.6	4.3–4.5
40	4.0–4.2	5.0–5.4
50	4.5–4.8	5.5–6.0

The heart rate and blood pressure changes in this study were similar to those when the drug was given intermittently. There was a modest delay in recovery from anaesthesia, which may not be acceptable in circumstances where adequate staff are not available.

The cardiovascular effects in these patients are of interest in that again the patients who received pancuronium (Fig. 5.3) showed a greater rise in mean arterial blood pressure and in heart rate than those given tubocurarine or in those patients breathing spontaneously.

During the study of ketamine infusion, an opportunity arose to test the hypothesis as to whether patients who have a known tolerance to alcohol are resistant to ketamine. A 35-year-old, 60 kg, man who had a known excessive alcohol intake required 875 mg ketamine over a 25-minute period.

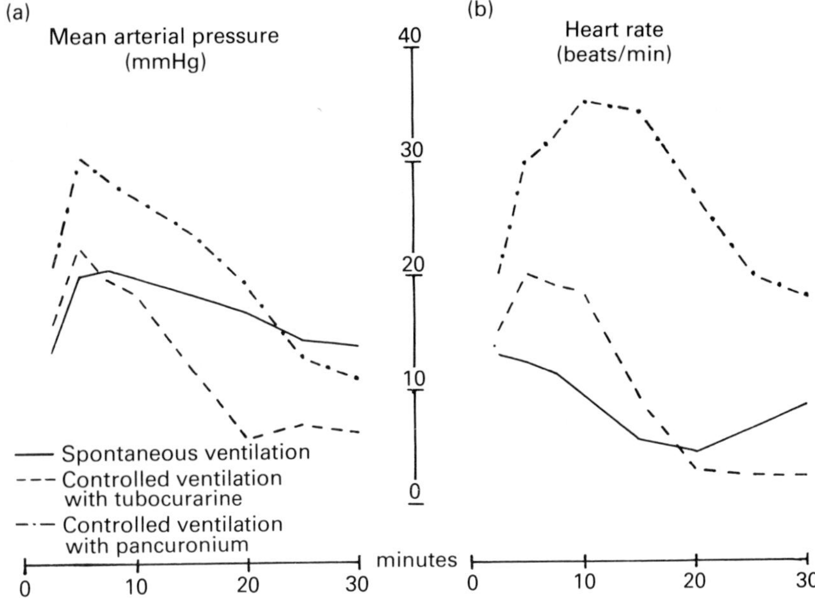

Fig. 5.3 Mean increase in mean arterial pressure (a) and heart rate (b) in patients anaesthetized with ketamine infusion.

This amounted to just over 14 mg·kg^{-1} as compared with the average requirement of in the region of 3—4 mg·kg^{-1}. Not only did this alcoholic patient show a resistance to ketamine but also the quality of anaesthesia was very unsatisfactory. It would appear from these observations that such patients constitute a contraindication to the use of ketamine infusions.

These results do not justify the use of ketamine infusion anaesthesia to the exclusion of other well established methods but they demonstrate the feasibility of such techniques and the approximate dose of ketamine required.

Organ toxicity

At the present time a note of caution should be sounded in relation to ketamine infusions, particularly in major surgery. We have noted changes in serum enzymes suggestive of liver dysfunction in some of the patients in this study; it has occurred to a greater extent than in a control series not receiving ketamine. Perhaps the use of 100 per cent oxygen may have played some part in the liver dysfunction revealed, and this is under investigation. The doses of ketamine employed were in the region of 3.5—4.0 mg·kg^{-1} for operations lasting 25—35 minutes.

Personal assessment (JWD)

For a drug which has as high an incidence of side effects as this to be continued to be used more than 10 years after its introduction into clinical practice is quite remarkable. There are those who feel that if it were no longer available then it would not be missed, but perhaps this is unfair, as it certainly has some unique properties. It will remain within the province of a few departments to continue investigations concerning its sequelae and one can only hope that within a reasonable time the 'taming' of this interesting agent will be complete.

As mentioned previously, although we have used ketamine in over 4000 administrations, no patient has suffered from any detectable ill effects due to a rise in blood pressure. Provided one remembers the well recognized contraindications to its use — hypertension, history of cardiovascular accident, psychiatric upset — our experience suggests that its dangers are less than originally thought.

References

Carson, I. W., Moore, J., Balmer, J. P., Dundee, J. W. and McNabb, T. G. (1973). Laryngeal competence with ketamine and other drugs. *Anesthesiology* **38,** 128—33.

Corssen, G. and Domino, E. F. (1966). Dissociative anesthesia: further pharmacologic studies and first clinical experience with the phencyclidine derivative CI 581. *Anesthesia and Analgesia . . . Current Researches* **45,** 29.

Domino, E. F., Chodoff, P. and Corssen, G. (1965). Pharmacologic effects of CI 581, a new dissociative anesthetic in man. *Clinical Pharmacology and Therapeutics* **6,** 279—90.

Dundee, J. W. and Lilburn, J. K. (1978). Ketamine-lorazepam: attenuation of psychic sequelae of ketamine by lorazepam. *Anaesthesia* **33,** 312—14.

Dundee, J. W., Lilburn, J. K. and Moore, J. (1978). Attempted reduction of the cardiostimulatory effects of ketamine by labetalol. *Anaesthesia* **33,** 506—11.

French, J. D., Verzeano, M. and Magoun, H. W. (1953). A neural basis of the anesthetic state. *Archives of Neurology and Psychiatry* **69,** 519—29.

Gibbs, J. M. (1977). A trial of ketamine anesthesia during abdominal surgery. In: *Clinical Use of Ketamine in Intravenous Drip Infusion,* Selected Proceedings of the Sixth World Congress of Anaesthesiology, Mexico City, April 24—30 1976, pp. 41—3. Excerpta Medica, Amsterdam.

Iwatsuki, K., Aoba, Y., Sato, K. and Iwatsuki, N. (1967). Clinical study on CI 581, a phencyclidine derivative. *Tohoku Journal of Experimental Medicine* **93,** 39—48.

Johnstone, M. (1972). The prevention of ketamine dreams. *Anaesthesia and Intensive Care* **1,** 70—4.

Johnstone, M. (1976). The cardiovascular effects of ketamine in man. *Anaesthesia* **31,** 873—82.

King, C. H. and Stephen, C. R. (1967). A new intravenous or intramuscular anesthetic. *Anesthesiology* **28,** 258.

Knox, J. W. D., Bovill, J. G., Clarke, R. S. J. and Dundee, J. W. (1970). Clinical studies of induction agents. XXXVI: Ketamine. *British Journal of Anaesthesia* **42,** 875—85.

Lilburn, J. K., Dundee, J. W. and Moore, J. (1978). Ketamine infusions: observations on technique, dosage and cardiovascular effects. *Anaesthesia* **33,** 315—21.

Lilburn, J. K., Moore, J. and Dundee, J. W. (1978). Attempts to attenuate the cardiostimulatory effects of ketamine. *Anaesthesia* **33,** 499—501.

Lilburn, J. K., Dundee, J. W., Nair, S. G., Fee, J. P. H. and Johnston, H. M. L. (1978). Ketamine sequelae: evaluation of the ability of various premedicants to attenuate its psychic action. *Anaesthesia* **33,** 307—11.

Morgan, M., Loh, L., Singer, L. and Moore, P. H. (1971). Ketamine as sole anaesthetic agent for minor surgical procedures. *Anaesthesia* **26,** 158—65.

Moruzzi, G. and Magoun, H. W. (1949). Brain stem reticular system and activation of the EEG. *Electroencephalography and Clinical Neurophysiology* **1,** 455—73.

Sabathie, M., Seguier, F., Fabre, P., Delperier, A., Bonnet, M. and Teychonneau, D. (1977). Ketamine hydrochloride in intravenous infusion for visceral surgery. In: *Clinical Use of Ketamine in Intravenous Drip Infusion,* Selected Proceedings of the Sixth World Congress of Anaesthesiology, Mexico City, April 24—30 1976, pp. 44—6. Excerpta Medica, Amsterdam.

Taylor, P. A. and Towey, R. M. (1971). Depression of laryngeal reflexes during ketamine anaesthesia. *British Medical Journal* **2,** 688—9.

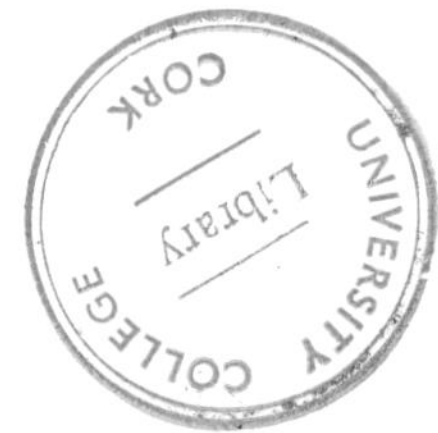

6

Etomidate

Etomidate is an intravenous hypnotic synthesized in the Belgian laboratories of Janssen Pharmaceutica at Beerse. It is a completely new type of anaesthetic, chemically unrelated to any commercially available agent.[1] The initial studies of its pharmacology and clinical use were carried out by Doenicke and his colleagues from the Surgical Polyclinic in Munich.[2–5]

Originally known as R 26490, in two Belgian publications it is referred to by its proprietary name, Hypnomidate.[6,7] At the time of writing (March 1978) etomidate is not available for routine clinical use, nor is there any clear evidence that it may be released in Britain. However, it has been widely studied — mostly in continental Europe and by members of the Belfast Department of Anaesthetics. Our findings, based on about 1400 administrations, are as yet unpublished and some of them will be included here.

This chapter differs from the others in that it is a comprehensive review of the current knowledge of a new drug. (For this reason the reference system is not in keeping with that of the rest of the book.)

Chemistry and physical properties

The chemical name of etomidate is *R*-(+)-ethyl-1-(1-phenyl ethyl)-1H-imidazole-5-carboxylate sulphate. Its structural formula is shown in Fig. 6.1 and its empirical formula is $C_{14}H_{16}N_2O_2,H_2SO_4$. Only the dextro isomer is anaesthetically active.[8]

It is a white crystalline powder with a molecular weight of 342.4. The salt is very soluble in water, but unstable in aqueous solution. The base is very soluble in propylene glycol and ethanol, freely soluble in polyethylene glycol and chloroform, sparingly soluble in acetone and water, and practically insoluble in ether and n-hexane.

Presentation

Although it is freely soluble in water, because of pain on injection two preparations in organic solvents have been studied. The constituents and some properties of these are given in Table 6.1 (we can offer no explanation for the differences in the two sets of pH values). Most of the continental European publications were with aqueous solutions, but it has not as yet been decided which formulation is to be made available for clinical use.

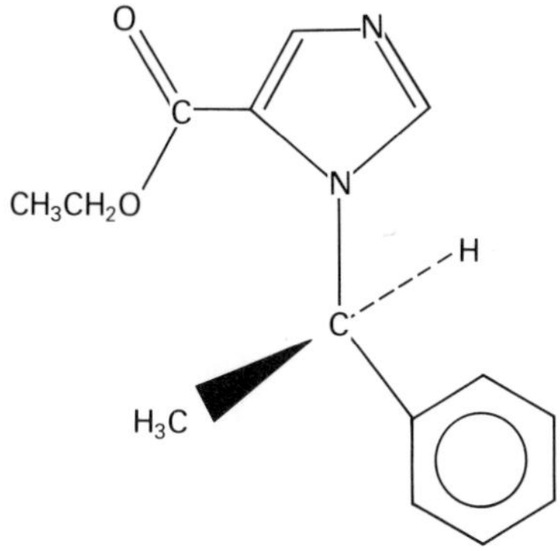

Fig. 6.1 Etomidate.

Once constituted, the aqueous solution should be used within 24 hours as it may lose its potency. The polyethylene glycol formulation has been available since 1976; it is dispensed in 5 ml ampoules of 0.2 per cent solution and is stable at room temperature. The polyethylene glycol solvent has a narrow range of molecular weight in the region of 3000. However, since it may be immunologically active and also is a possible cause of haemolysis, its use has been suspended. The propylene glycol formulation is the currently available form of the drug. It is dispensed in 10 ml ampoules of 0.2 per cent solution. There is no problem with the stability of this preparation, which can be left at room temperature for over two years.

Table 6.1 Some properties of the different formulations of etomidate

Solvent		$mg \cdot ml^{-1}$	pH at 37°C		Osmolarity (b) ($mmol \cdot kg^{-1}$)	Viscosity (a) ($Ns \cdot m^{-2}$)
			(a)	(b)		
Water*	(Aqueous)	0.15	3.2	3.46	254	0.08
Polyethylene glycol	(PEG)	0.20	4.5	5.21	550	0.40
Propylene glycol	(PG)	0.20	6.0	8.10	4640	0.25

(a) our estimation (b) Hendry, Miller and Lees[9]
*Containing phosphate buffer

Onset of action and potency

Etomidate is a rapidly acting drug in effective doses, causing unconsciousness in one arm—brain circulation time.[10,11] Figure 6.2 is our findings with onset of sleep, as judged by the time when the patient stops counting following the administration of varying doses of the propylene glycol preparation injected as quickly as possible at the height of reactive hyperaemia of the forearm.[12] This is based on 110 observations and it will be seen that sleep occurred in an extremely short time with high doses — apparently shorter than one arm—brain circulation time. This anomaly is due to the viscosity of the solution, since the onset time was measured from the end of the injection; doses of 0.3—0.4 mg·kg^{-1} may require 10—12 ml solution and take 5—6 seconds to inject. However, there is no doubt that etomidate is a rapidly acting drug and this agrees with the clinical impression of all workers. We cannot comment on the statement that a faster injection produces a quicker onset[5] and *vice versa*.[10] Kay has noted that the onset of action of etomidate is as rapid as that of methohexitone.[13]

The relative potency of induction agents is difficult to assess.[12] From the individual cases in Fig. 6.2 it was possible to calculate that the minimum dose of etomidate which would consistently result in the onset of anaesthesia in 10—10.5 seconds was 0.25 mg·kg^{-1}. Comparing this with similar data for

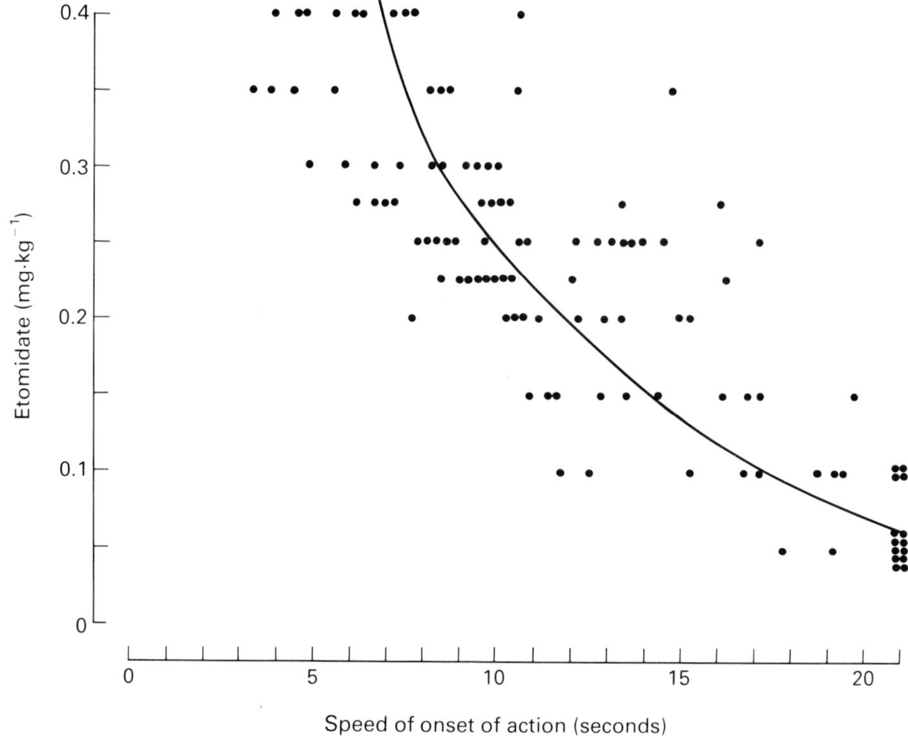

Fig. 6.2 Individual (•) and mean (curve) time of onset of anaesthesia following varying doses of etomidate in propylene glycol. Time was measured from end of injection until the patient stopped counting, using the method of Clarke and his colleagues.[12]

other drugs[12] it is estimated that, on a weight for weight basis, etomidate is approximately four times more potent than methohexitone and twelve times more potent than thiopentone.

Fate in the body

There is a paucity of published work on the pharmacokinetics of etomidate and only the findings of Heykants and his co-workers[8,14] are relevant. It is heavily (78 per cent) bound to plasma albumin, whereas only 60 per cent of its metabolites are bound; 3 per cent is bound to globulin. It enters the brain quickly and, like thiopentone, leaves it rapidly due to redistribution in the body. The fast component of the plasma decay curve has a half-life of 1.2 minutes. Much of the active drug is distributed to muscle and fat.

Etomidate is rapidly broken down, being mainly hydrolysed by esterases, both in the liver and plasma.[5,8,14] Plasma levels decrease rapidly over the first half hour, less rapidly for the next 3½ hours and more slowly thereafter. As with thiopentone, disappearance from the plasma occurs in three phases[15] and detectable amounts of etomidate persist in plasma for at least 6 hours.[16]

Tritium-labelled etomidate sulphate was used in the study of Heykants and colleagues.[8] They found that the main (80 per cent) metabolite is *R*-(+)-(α methylbenzyl)-5-imidazol carboxylic acid (R 28141), which is pharmacologically inactive. A number of other metabolites are also formed by a process of decarboxylation and oxidative dealkylation and may include glucuronides. There is a rapid build-up of the metabolites for 30 minutes and thereafter they decline slowly. Inhibition of the esterase *in vitro* by potassium fluoride keeps the etomidate unchanged in plasma for several months; this confirms the involvement of esterases in its metabolism.[16]

Of the total administered drug, 87 per cent is excreted in the urine (3 per cent of which is in an unchanged form) and 13 per cent in the bile.[8]

Clinical effects

Injection pain

Pain on injection is a distinct disadvantage of etomidate and has been noted by many workers[10,11,13,17,18] who have given incidences ranging from 10 to 63 per cent. Variations in observers, dosage, rate of injection, site, size of vein, preanaesthetic medication and formulation are factors which may influence the incidence, and these have not been standardized in the different studies.

From our cases, we have selected patients undergoing a standard operation (minor gynaecology) and divided these into groups, each of 20—30 patients, according to:

1. Preanaesthetic medication:
   (a) nil;
   (b) diazepam 10 mg;
   (c) pethidine 75 mg.

2. Rate of injection:
   (a) slow: 1 mg·s^{-1};
   (b) fast: 2 mg·s^{-1}.
3. Formulation used.

The findings (Fig. 6.3) show an incidence range from 10 to 50 per cent in different groups. Because of the comparability of the size of the groups these can be pooled to give an overall percentage as shown in Table 6.2. A slow rate of injection was a significant factor in the incidence of pain ($P<0.05$), which was significantly higher with the aqueous as compared with the other two formulations ($P<0.025$). Pethidine premedication reduced the frequency of complaints of injection pain as compared with unpremedicated patients ($P<0.05$).

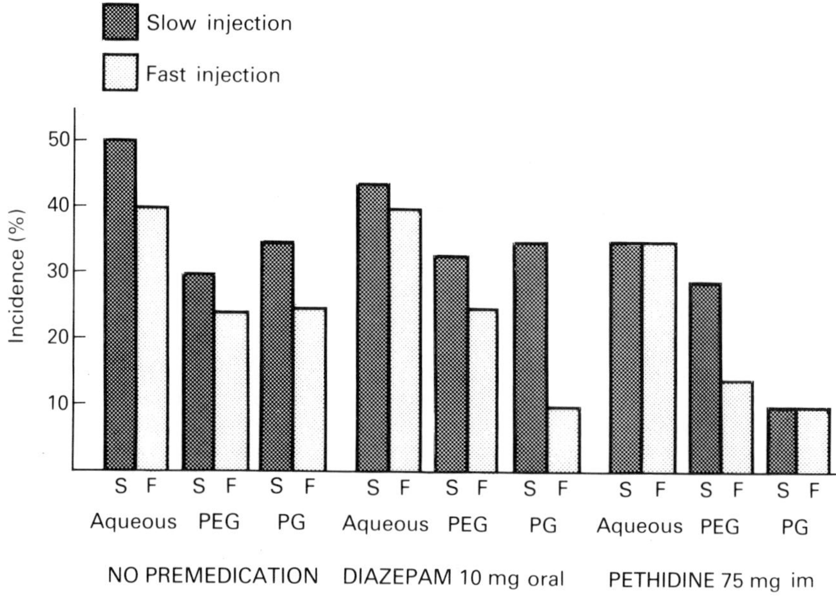

Fig. 6.3 Percentage incidence of pain on injection following 0.3 mg·kg^{-1} etomidate injected at either 1 mg·s^{-1} (slow) or 2 mg·s^{-1} (fast) in aqueous, polyethylene glycol (PEG) or propylene glycol (PG) solutions in patients given the premedicants shown.

As shown in Table 6.2, the site of injection and size of vein are also important factors. Pain occurs most frequently from injections given into small veins and in the wrist or back of hand.

These findings in relation to the speed of injection,[11,13] preanaesthetic medication,[11] and site and size of vein[13,19] are in agreement with those of other workers. Pain is also reduced when the injection is made into a rapidly running infusion.[20] Kay[13] has reported that a preparation of etomidate in cremophor is followed by a low incidence of injection pain, but we have not had an opportunity of using this formulation. To put these findings into perspective, it should be noted that pain rarely occurs with thiopentone injections and in 8—17 per cent of patients given methohexitone.[18,21]

Kay[13] has attempted to reduce injection pain by combining etomidate with lignocaine, but this was not very effective.

Table 6.2 Factors influencing pain on injection

Variable factors		Incidence of pain (%)
Rate of injection	Slow speed	34
	Fast speed	25
Premedication	None	33
	Diazepam	32
	Pethidine	22
Formulation	Aqueous	41
	PEG	26
	PG	22
Site of injection	Antecubital	22
	Forearm	29
	Wrist	48
	Back of hand	51
Size of vein	Large	24
	Moderate	41
	Small	81

Excitatory effects

The most important problem with etomidate is the high incidence of spontaneous involuntary muscle movement, tremor and hypertonus following induction.[3,10,11,13,15,17,22,23] The reported incidence (5—80 per cent) has varied because due account has not always been taken of factors which are known to influence this complication with other intravenous anaesthetics.

We have examined the incidence of excitatory effects in the patients in whom we studied pain on injection. Figure 6.4 shows that preanaesthetic medication is an important factor. Compared with unpremedicated patients, diazepam reduces the incidence significantly ($P<0.0005$), while pethidine has an even more marked protective effect ($P<0.0001$). Table 6.3 shows our findings in 1400 patients, in which the speed of injection is not taken into account. The incidences are similar to those in Fig. 6.4 except that, with the larger number of cases, the propylene glycol formulation now causes a significantly higher incidence than the other two preparations ($P<0.0005$).

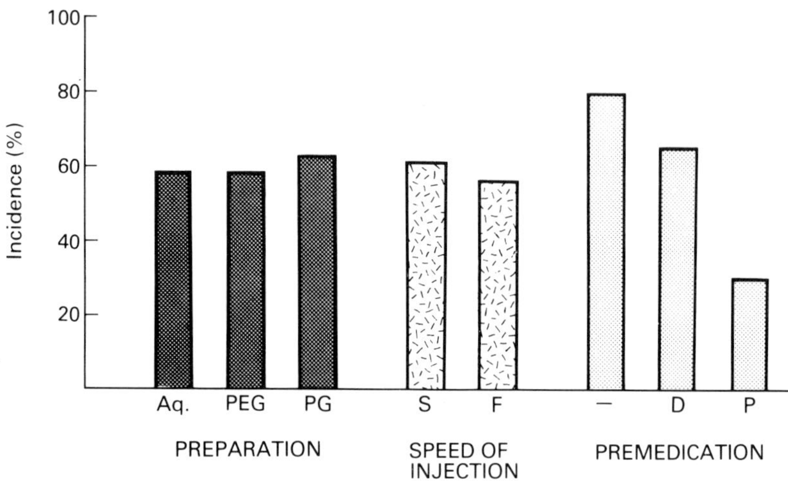

Fig. 6.4 Percentage incidence of excitatory effects following 0.3 mg·kg^{-1} etomidate. Aq., aqueous; PEG, polyethylene glycol; PG, propylene glycol; S, slow; F, fast; D, diazepam; P, pethidine.

In contrast to Fig. 6.4, there are several continental European reports of series of patients in which muscle movements have not been noted as a major drawback. In these the etomidate was preceded by intravenous fentanyl. This produces an effect similar to pethidine premedication.

Again one has to put these data into perspective. In unpremedicated patients the incidence of excitatory effects following 4—5 mg·kg^{-1} thiopentone is about 8 per cent[24,25] and about 30 per cent with methohexitone.[24] With opiate premedication this is reduced to 5—6 per cent for both drugs. The incidence with methohexitone in patients premedicated with diazepam is in the region of 25—30 per cent.[26,27] Clearly etomidate causes a much higher incidence of excitatory effects than the two standard barbiturates.

Not only is the incidence of excitatory effects greater with etomidate but the severity of these effects is also greater than with barbiturates. On occasion, marked hypertonus may interfere with positioning of the unpremedicated patient, as occurs with ketamine.

Table 6.3 Percentage incidence of excitatory effects following etomidate in 1400 patients, grouped according to the formulation and premedication used

Formulation	No premedication	Benzodiazepines	Opiates
Aqueous	66	64	44
Polyethylene glycol	67	59	34
Propylene glycol	81	76	28

Respiratory complications

In unpremedicated patients, induction doses of etomidate are followed by an incidence of cough and hiccough which is similar to that with methohexitone. The overall incidence in our study was 21 per cent, compared with 26 per cent with methohexitone.[24] Cough and hiccough are of short duration and do not interfere with the course of anaesthesia. In our study the frequency of this side effect was reduced by premedication with diazepam (to 12 per cent), and with pethidine (to 9 per cent). Respiratory complications seem to occur most frequently in patients who exhibit muscle movements. It appears probable that the excitatory effects also involve the diaphragm. Severe laryngospasm is very uncommon after etomidate.

There are conflicting reports on the incidence of apnoea after etomidate.[9,10,11,13,15,23] We have not found respiratory depression to be a clinically significant problem in unpremedicated patients or in those given diazepam. It occurred in about 1 in 20 of all patients receiving the drug in all these groups. In contrast, as expected, the incidence was much higher (10—15 per cent) in patients premedicated with pethidine. Arterial oxygen content remains within normal limits during anaesthesia.[3,28]

Cardiovascular effects

Lack of cardiovascular toxicity is said to be one of the outstanding features of etomidate[2,4,7,10,11,22,29,30,31,32,33,39,40] — without such claims it is unlikely that clinical trials would have gone so far. Data on this will be reviewed in some detail.

The initial investigations[1] showed that etomidate had minimal effects on the cardiovascular system in rats. In subsequent studies[34] Janssen and his colleagues found that it had less effect than comparable doses of propanidid or thiopentone. Microelectrode techniques have shown that it is devoid of depressant effect on the spontaneous activity of atrial muscle and does not alter conduction in Purkinje fibre.[35] Although etomidate in doses of 1.25 and 2.5 $mg \cdot kg^{-1}$ decreased blood pressure in the intact dog, it had no effect on dp/dt_{max} in man (at a constant heart rate of $120 \cdot min^{-1}$) or on mean aortic and coronary blood flow.[36] The only other animal work is that of Weymar and his colleagues,[37] who confirmed the lack of direct cardiovascular toxicity of etomidate. Cardiac output was not depressed because of a slight increase in heart rate.

There have been many clinical studies with etomidate and, in general, these have confirmed the low cardiovascular toxicity.[33] In fit patients, Bruckner and his colleagues[38,40] found that 0.3 $mg \cdot kg^{-1}$ produced a slight increase in cardiac index, accompanied by a slight fall in heart rate, a slight fall in arterial pressure (14 per cent) and peripheral resistance (17 per cent); dp/dt_{max} rose (9 per cent) with maximum effects occurring about three minutes after injection. They considered changes to be small in comparison with the effects of other intravenous anaesthetics and quote the unpublished findings of Jaganeau and his colleagues in support of this.

In a comprehensive comparative study, Kettler and Sonntag[29] investigated coronary blood flow and myocardial oxygen consumption (MVO_2) in healthy patients. Increases in heart rate are, in the main, responsible for the increases in MVO_2 which were found with propanidid (+ 82 per cent), ketamine (+ 78 per cent), Althesin (+ 63 per cent), thiopentone (+ 55 per cent) and methohexitone (+ 44 per cent). In contrast, etomidate did not produce significant changes in MVO_2. Coronary arteriovenous difference was not significantly altered by any of the agents and etomidate alone seemed to have a true, but weak, coronary vasodilator effect. In another study[22] the same group of workers gave an induction dose of 0.3 $mg \cdot kg^{-1}$ etomidate followed by an infusion of 0.12 $mg \cdot kg \cdot min^{-1}$; they found that coronary blood flow was increased by 19 per cent and coronary resistance decreased 19 per cent, leaving a constant coronary perfusion pressure.

In clinical doses etomidate reduces peripheral vascular resistance[29,39] with increases of as much as 60 per cent in blood flow. This action may be potentiated by other drugs.[17,22,33] Although van Aken and Rolly[41] found that cerebral blood flow was significantly reduced in most regions of the brain by etomidate, Lazarevic and colleagues[42] found no alteration in intracranial pressure in hydrocephalic patients.

Our own cardiovascular studies are limited to blood pressure and heart rate readings. We found that normal induction doses cause effects which are similar to those of methohexitone[23,43] without the marked tachycardia which the barbiturate causes. Even after large single doses of 0.9 $mg \cdot kg^{-1}$ hypotension was not a problem.

Histamine release

Unlike other intravenous anaesthetics, etomidate does not release significant amounts of histamine.[5,36] As supporting evidence for this Doenicke[5] found a steady basophil count during anaesthesia. However, there are reports of rashes occurring in varying parts of the body (mainly head, neck and upper trunk) following etomidate.[6,18,19] We found a very low incidence (3 in 1400) of rashes. However, in our series, one woman having repeat administrations of etomidate—suxamethonium for electroconvulsive therapy developed a marked generalized rash each time the drug was given. The propylene glycol formulation was used and the rash occurred immediately on injection before any other drugs were given. She showed no other evidence of histamine release and had no bronchospasm or hypotension.

Anaesthetic action

This should, of course, include excitatory and other side effects but for the present discussion is limited to its effects on the electroencephalogram, the duration of action and cumulative effects.

The e.e.g. pattern of anaesthesia with etomidate is similar to that of barbiturates and propanidid.[44,45] Despite the induction complications, on the whole patients find etomidate anaesthesia to be pleasant and we have encountered very few who would not be prepared to have it on a second occasion.

Kay[46] studied its cumulative effect by repeating doses of 0.1 mg·kg^{-1} as required to maintain sleep and found a linear relationship between dose and duration of sleep over the rate of 0.1—1.4 mg·kg^{-1}. (In his paper he gave the range as 1—8 mg·kg^{-1}, but clearly this is an error for 0.1—0.8, otherwise a 50 kg patient would need 267 ml of the aqueous or 200 ml of the propylene glycol solution over 25 minutes.) This linear relationship is similar to that found with propanidid,[47] G 29 505[48] and Althesin.[49] It is much less cumulative than thiopentone.

Kay[46] has compared mean waking and late recovery times, as judged by Hannington-Kiff's ocular test,[50] with three doses of etomidate (0.1, 0.2, 0.4 mg·kg^{-1} and 1.5 mg·kg^{-1} methohexitone (Fig. 6.5). This shows a linear relationship over the dose range studied. It also suggests that delayed recovery is more prolonged after methohexitone than with etomidate. The ratio of time to waking and late recovery averaged 1:2.75 for 0.2 mg·kg^{-1} etomidate and 1:3.39 for 1.5 mg·kg^{-1} methohexitone.

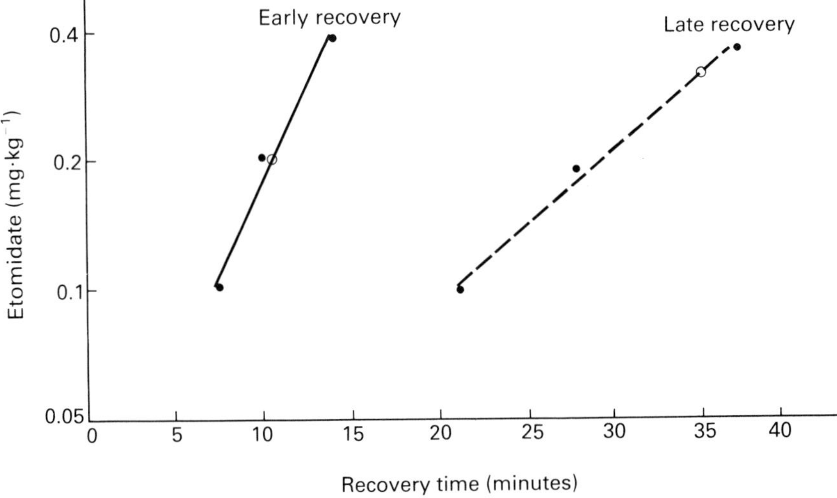

Fig. 6.5 Recovery, early and late, from three doses of etomidate • and 1.5 mg methohexitone o. (From Kay, 1976[46].)

Figure 6.6 is unpublished findings of a study involving 9 groups each of 10 unpremedicated adult patients given doses of etomidate over the range of 0.05—0.9 mg·kg^{-1}. The duration of sleep was taken as the time until the patient opened his eyes on command. Only 1 patient lost consciousness with the lowest dose and 8 out of 10 with 0.1 mg·kg^{-1}. There was a linear relationship (r = +0.97) over the dose range studied, with no evidence of a proportionately longer effect from the higher dose. In contrast with several other intravenous anaesthetics, the end point of recovery was always abrupt and easily defined with etomidate, even after large doses.

The findings of our study and that of Kay[46] would suggest that the duration of anaesthesia with etomidate is similar to that with equivalent doses of methohexitone, and recovery is definitely quicker than from thiopentone. Although there is no scientific evidence to support this statement, one gets the impression that early recovery probably occurs more rapidly with etomidate than with Althesin. In contrast with the barbiturates, complete recovery is probably more rapid with the steroid or etomidate.

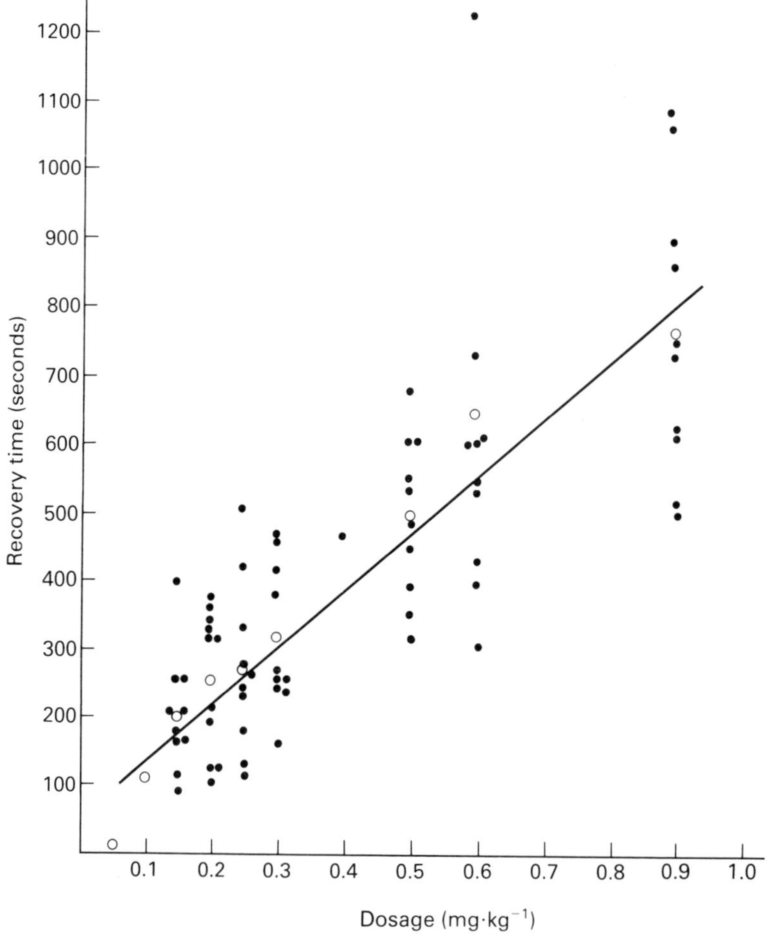

Fig. 6.6 Average (o) and individual (•) durations of sleep (taken as time from end of injection until the patient opens eyes on command) in groups of 10 patients given differing doses of etomidate.

Interaction with suxamethonium

Early in the clinical evaluation of etomidate an impression was formed that suxamethonium was less effective when given with this agent than after the barbiturates. Bruckner and his colleagues[38] had made a similar comment based on finding an inadequate degree of relaxation when 1.2 mg·kg^{-1} suxamethonium was given with etomidate.

Using the method employed in studying interactions between suxamethonium and barbiturates or eugenols,[51] the average duration of respiratory depression (based on clinical observations) and apnoea following 50 mg suxamethonium was studied. Table 6.4 shows the findings in 100 patients induced with etomidate (0.3 mg·kg^{-1}) and 40 with thiopentone (5 mg·kg^{-1}). There was little difference in the duration of apnoea with the two induction agents but, on the average, respiratory depression lasted significantly longer in those patients induced with thiopentone ($P<0.02$). It is doubtful if this difference is of great clinical significance, although we have found some problems when etomidate-suxamethonium was used for bronchoscopy with the apnoeic-ventilation technique. Similar problems have arisen with electroconvulsive therapy.

Table 6.4 Average duration (± sem) and range of apnoea and respiratory depression (seconds) after 50 mg suxamethonium in an unselected group of patients

	Etomidate (0.15%)	Thiopentone (2.5%)
Apnoea:		
Duration	178 ± 7	194 ± 17
Range	0–530	0–480
Respiratory depression:		
Duration	250 ± 9	300 ± 20
Range	90–625	145–630

Sequelae

Recovery from etomidate is usually smooth and it is free from ketamine-like effects.

We have found a significantly higher incidence of vomiting and nausea in the first six hours after operation in unpremedicated patients anaesthetized with etomidate-nitrous oxide-oxygen as compared with a similar series[24] induced with methohexitone or thiopentone. This information (Table 6.5) was obtained from women undergoing minor gynaecological operations of similar duration who were not given any other drugs. Almost all of this sickness occurred during the first hour after operation. In further studies we did not find a higher incidence of sickness when pethidine premedication was given; this surprising finding agrees with that of Holdcroft and colleagues.[19]

Without giving supporting evidence or comparison with the effects of other drugs, many workers have commented on the low incidence of venous

Table 6.5 Percentage incidence of emetic sequelae during the first 6 hours of anaesthesia in unpremedicated patients receiving etomidate, methohexitone and thiopentone for minor gynaecological procedures

	Vomiting	Nausea
Formulation of etomidate:		
Aqueous	30	13
Propylene glycol	26	21
Polyethylene glycol	33	15
Methohexitone	15	12
Thiopentone	13	6

sequelae. It has even been claimed that no damage occurs to arterial or venous walls.[30] We have made a comparison of venous sequelae with the three preparations of etomidate, using a standard injection technique and follow-up.[52] No other drug or infusion was given through the vein nor was a tourniquet applied. Table 6.6 shows that the propylene glycol preparation is followed by a very high incidence of venous sequelae and that all preparations cause a slightly higher incidence than thiopentone or methohexitone. There is some evidence to suggest that rapid injection may result in a slightly higher incidence of venous sequelae from etomidate. The effect is related to dosage; an overall incidence of 13 per cent sequelae was found with 0.3 $mg \cdot kg^{-1}$ rising to 37 per cent with doses in excess of 0.9 $mg \cdot kg^{-1}$.

Table 6.6 Comparison of the incidence of venous thrombosis found on the 2nd or 3rd day following various formulations of etomidate with published data on thiopentone, methohexitone[53] and Althesin[54] using similar methodology

Drug	Formulation	No. patients	Incidence (%)
Etomidate	Aqueous	227	10.6
	PEG	104	7.7
	PG	179	23.4
Thiopentone	2.5%	202	2.0
	5%	307	5.8
Methohexitone	1%	203	3.0
	2%	251	6.3
Althesin		330	3.0

Other effects

One of the initial animal studies which recommended that etomidate merited study in man[34] showed it to have a very high therapeutic index of 26.4 as compared with 6.7 for propanidid and 9.5 for methohexitone. It was also shown to have minimal toxicity on repeated administration and to be free from teratogenic effects.

Apart from a rise in serum potassium in patients in whom myoclonic movements were marked,[19] there is nothing to suggest that etomidate causes any biochemical changes in the body.

In view of the possible interaction between etomidate and suxamethonium, the plasma cholinesterase level was measured in 21 patients before and 2, 10 and 60 minutes after etomidate (without suxamethonium). Butyrylthiocholine was used as the substrate in the colorimetric method employed. There was a progressive fall in the average cholinesterase level during the study period (Fig. 6.7), the changes being statistically significant at 60 minutes (using the paired 't' test); however, all changes fell within the known range of error of the method employed and are probably of no clinical significance.

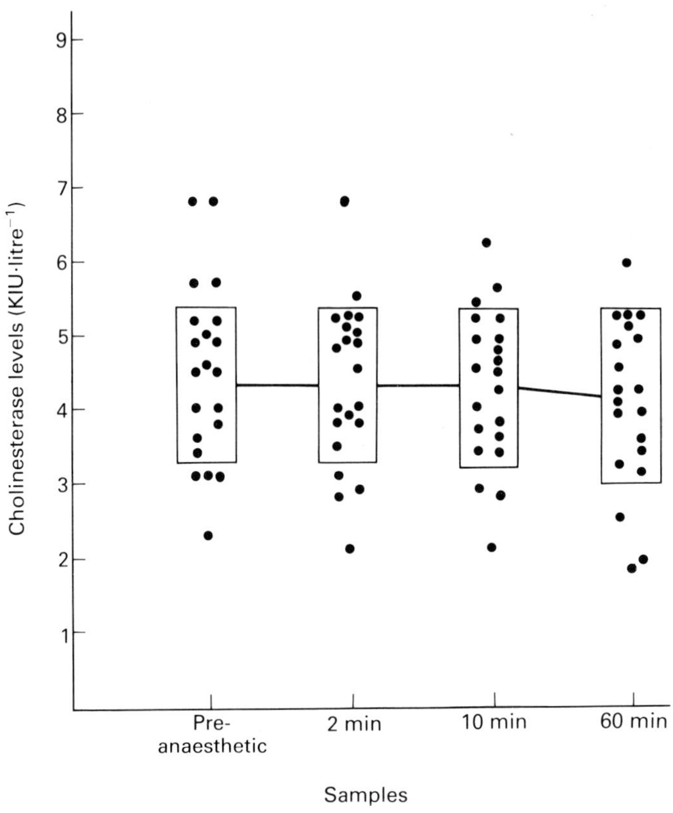

Fig. 6.7 Individual and average ± SD cholinesterase readings before and at 2, 10 and 60 minutes after 0.3–0.6 mg·kg^{-1} etomidate. Cholinesterase levels are expressed in international units (IU) per litre, the normal range being 3000–9300 (3–9.3 KIU) at 25°C.

In the light of its potential use in large doses for infusion and the possible dangers of this,[55] liver function studies were carried out in 20 healthy patients undergoing minor operations averaging 12 minutes in duration and given an average dose of 1.2 $mg \cdot kg^{-1}$ etomidate. The tests with the normal range (international units per litre) were:

Table 6.7

	Normal range (Ul^{-1})	SD of the method (Ul^{-1})
1. Aspartate aminotransferase (AST)	10–40	7
2. Alanine aminotransferase (ALT)	10–45	7
3. Alkaline phosphatase (AP)	35–105	6
4. Gamma glutamyl transpeptidase (γGT)	5–22	6
5. Plasma cholinesterase (ChE)	50–110 Michel units	3 Michel units

These were carried out preoperatively and on the 3rd to 4th and 13th to 15th postoperative days.

Figure 6.8 gives the average readings. This shows no evidence of a hepatotoxic action of large doses of etomidate. No comparable study of liver function has been published.

There is no published study on kidney function during etomidate anaesthesia. Tarnow and his colleagues[56] found a slight decrease in renal blood flow with a corresponding increase in vascular resistance. These changes were considered of no importance.

Clinical evaluation

In the light of what has already been stated, it is not surprising that some workers have commented on the poor quality of anaesthesia produced by etomidate. Perhaps more surprising was a statement by Doenicke[44] that he had experience of nearly 7000 administrations without any complications.

It is sufficient here to give our own data on the evaluation of the induction compared with similar observations by the same workers with other agents. Pooling all our data with standard induction doses, and ignoring beneficial effects of opiate premedication, we found:

Table 6.8

	Etomidate	Thiopentone	Methohexitone
Uneventful	26	78	51
Slight upset	46	18	32
Marked upset	17	4	13
Very troublesome	11	0	4

The thiopentone and methohexitone data were obtained in unpremedicated patients.[24] These figures indicate unequivocally the disadvantages of etomidate.

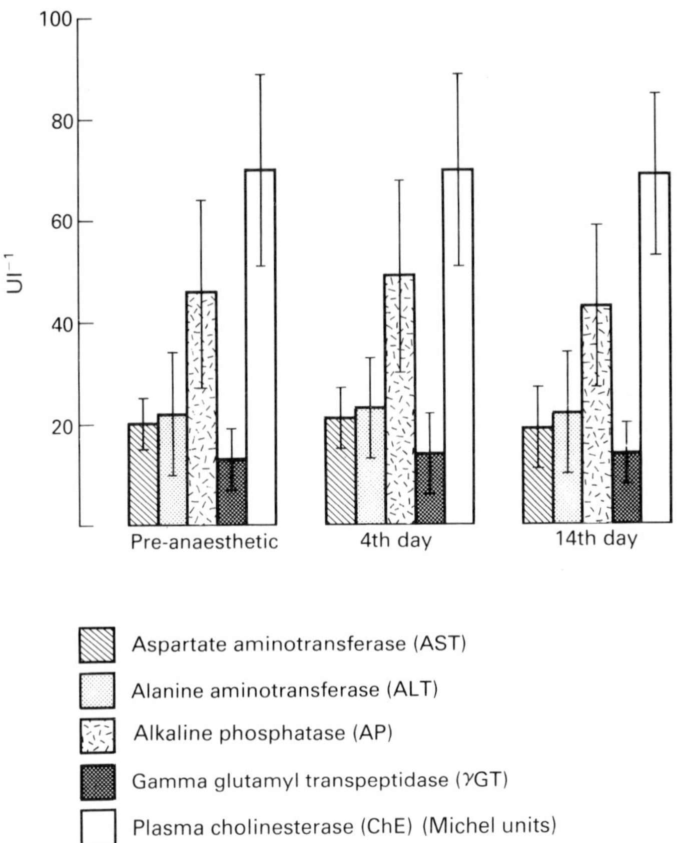

Fig. 6.8 Average and SD of five liver function tests carried out before, 3–4 days and 13–15 days after large doses of etomidate.

Personal assessment (JWD)

In making an assessment of the possible role of etomidate as an intravenous anaesthetic, one can state categorically that it cannot be equated with thiopentone or Althesin as regards smoothness of induction. As a straight induction agent it causes an unacceptably high incidence of side effects. Perhaps a different formulation may solve the problem of pain on injection and this may, in turn, reduce the excitatory effects, but this is for the future.

Accepting its inferiority as an induction agent, has it a role either in balanced anaesthesia, including neurolept (NLA), or as a continuous infusion? Perhaps its low cardiovascular toxicity could be exploited. In a balanced technique it would be acceptable when given immediately following fentanyl; such a combination of two short-acting drugs might be more rational than the droperidol—fentanyl mixture. This certainly is worth exploring, particularly in the fields of outpatient endoscopy, minor operations and perhaps even dentistry.

The absence of a cumulative effect makes it an attractive drug for continuous infusion. In this respect the absence of histamine release (and, it is hoped absence of hypersensitivity) makes it a suitable alternative to Althesin. The lack of demonstrable hepatotoxicity from very large doses is favourable for its use for continuous infusion.

An editorial in March 1976[57] commented: 'It may be stated . . . that etomidate is not the "ideal anaesthetic". However, at a time when some anaesthetists are exploring methods which lessen the need for gaseous anaesthetics, it merits further study.' This would seem to be a reasonable point of view, except that one year (and about 1000 more cases) later one still remains uncertain of its place as an intravenous anaesthetic.

References

1. Janssen, P. A. J., Niemegeers, C. J. E., Schellekens, K. H. L. and Lenaerts, F. M. (1971). Etomidate, *R*-(+)-ethyl-1-(α-methyl-benzyl) imidazole-5-carboxylate (R 16659), a potent short-acting and relatively atoxic intravenous hypnotic agent in rats. *Arzneimittel-Forschung* **21,** 1234—43.
2. Doenicke, A., Wagner, E. and Beetz, K. H. (1973). Blutgasanalysen (arteriell) nach drei kurzwirkenden i.v. Hypnotica (Propanidid, Etomidate und Methohexital). *Anaesthesist* **22,** 353—6.
3. Doenicke, A., Kugler, J., Penzel, G., Laub, M., Kalmar, L., Killian, I. and Bezecny, H. (1973). Hirnfunktion und Toleranzbriete nach Etomidate einem neuen barbituratfreien i.v. applizierbaren Hypnoticum. *Anaesthesist* **22,** 357.
4. Doenicke, A., Gabanyi, D., Lemcke, H. and Schurk-Bulich, M. (1974). Circulatory behaviour and myocardial function after the administration of three short-acting i.v. hypnotics, etomidate, propanidid and methohexital. *Anaesthesist* **23,** 108—15.
5. Doenicke, A., Lorenz, W., Beigl, R., Bezecny, H., Uhlig, G., Kalmar, L., Praetorius, B. and Mann, G. (1973). Histamine release after intravenous application of short-acting hypnotics. A comparison of etomidate, Althesin CT 1341 and propanidid. *British Journal of Anaesthesia* **45,** 1097—104.
6. Popescu, D. T. (1976). Clinical study of Althesin and hypnomidate. Proceedings of the Belgian Congress of Anesthesiology II, Brussels, 10—13 September 1975. *Acta anaesthesiologica Belgica* **27,** 196—207.

7. Popescu, D. T., Lazarevic, Z., Rejger, V. and Stamenkovic, L. (1976). Etomidate, cardiac performances in comparison with alphaxalone/alphadolone, thiopentone and neuroleptanaesthesia. *Abstract 187,* Sixth World Congress of Anaesthesiology, Mexico City, April 24—30, p. 92. Excerpta Medica, Amsterdam.
8. Heykants, J. J. P., Meuldermauf, W. E. G., Michiels, L. J. M., Lewi, P. J. and Janssen, P. A. J. (1975). Distribution, metabolism and excretion of etomidate, a short acting hypnotic drug, in the rat. Comparative study of (R)-(+) and (S)-(—) etomidate. *Archives internationales de pharmacodynamie et de thérapie* **216,** 113—29.
9. Hendry, J. G. B., Miller, B. M. and Lees, N. W. (1977). Etomidate in a new solvent. Clinical evaluation. *Anaesthesia* **32,** 996—9.
10. Morgan, M., Lumley, J. and Whitwam, J. G. (1975). Etomidate, a new water-soluble non-barbiturate intravenous induction agent. *Lancet* **i,** 955—6.
11. Gooding, J. M. and Corssen, G. (1976). Etomidate an ultra short acting non barbiturate agent for anesthesia induction. *Anesthesia and Analgesia . . . Current Researches* **55,** 286—9.
12. Clarke, R. S. J., Dundee, J. W., Barron, D. W., McArdle, L. and Howard, P. J. (1968). Clinical studies of induction agents. XXVI: Relative potencies of thiopentone, methohexitone and propanidid. *British Journal of Anaesthesia* **40,** 593—601.
13. Kay, B. (1976). A clinical assessment of the use of etomidate in children. *British Journal of Anaesthesia* **48,** 207—11.
14. Lewi, P. J., Heykants, J. J. P. and Janssen, P. A. J. (1976). Intravenous pharmacokinetic profile in rats of etomidate, a short-acting hypnotic drug. *Archives internationales de pharmacodynamie et de thérapie* **220,** 72—85.
15. Ghoneim, M. M., Van Hamme, M. J., Yamada, T. and Ambre, J. J. (1976). Etomidate: a clinical, electroencephalographic and pharmacokinetic comparison with thiopental. Paper presented at the Annual Meeting of the American Society of Anesthesiologists, October 11 1976.
16. Van Hamme, M. J., Ambre, J. J. and Ghoneim, M. M. (1977). Mass fragmentographic determination of plasma etomidate concentrations. *Journal of Pharmaceutical Sciences* **66,** 1344—6.
17. Dubois-Primo, J., Bastenier-Geens, J., Genicot, C. and Rucquoi, M. (1976). A comparative study of etomidate and methohexital, as induction agents for analgesic anesthesia. Proceedings of the Belgian Congress of Anesthesiology II, Brussels, 10—13 September 1975. *Acta anaesthesiologica Belgica* **27,** 187—95.
18. Doom, A. and Mundeleer, P. (1976). Etomidate and tonsillectomy. Proceedings of the Belgian Congress of Anesthesiology II, Brussels, 10—13 September 1975. *Acta anaesthesiologica Belgica* **27,** 181—6.
19. Holdcroft, A., Morgan, M., Whitwam, J. G. and Lumley, J. (1976). Effect of dose and premedication on induction complications with etomidate. *British Journal of Anaesthesia* **48,** 199—204.

20. Thomas, B., Meirlaen, L., Rolly, G. and Weyne, L. (1976). Clinical use of etomidate. Proceedings of the Belgian Congress of Anesthesiology II, Brussels, 10—13 September 1975. *Acta anaesthesiologica Belgica* **27,** 167—74.
21. Rowlands, D. E. (1969). Pain after methohexitone. *Anaesthesia* **24,** 289.
22. Kettler, D., Sonntag, H., Donath, U., Regensburger, D. and Schenk, H. D. (1974). Haemodynamics, myocardial function, oxygen requirement and oxygen supply of the human heart after the administration of etomidate. *Anaesthesist* **23,** 116—21.
23. Zacharias, M., Clarke, R. S. J., Dundee, J. W. and Johnston, S. B. (1978). An evaluation of three preparations of etomidate. *British Journal of Anaesthesia* **50,** 925—9.
24. Dundee, J. W. (1963). Clinical studies of induction agents. VII: A comparison of eight intravenous anaesthetics as main agents for a standard operation. *British Journal of Anaesthesia* **35,** 784—94.
25. Barron, D. W., Dundee, J. W., Gilmore, W. R. and Howard, P. J. (1966). Clinical studies of induction agents. XVI: A comparison of thiopentone, buthalitone, hexobarbitone and thiamylal. *British Journal of Anaesthesia* **38,** 802—11.
26. Haslett, W. H. K. and Dundee, J. W. (1968). Studies of drugs given before anaesthesia. XIV: Two benzodiazepine derivatives, chlordiazepoxide and diazepam. *British Journal of Anaesthesia* **40,** 250—8.
27. Assaf, R. A. E., Dundee, J. W. and Gamble, J. A. S. (1975). The influence of the route of administration on the clinical action of diazepam. *Anaesthesia* **30,** 152—8.
28. Hempelmann, G., Piepenbrock, S., Hempelmann, W. and Karliczek, G. (1974). Influence of Althesine and etomidate on blood gases (continuous pO_2-monitoring) and haemodynamics in man. *Acta anaesthesiologica Belgica* **25,** 402—12.
29. Kettler, D. and Sonntag, H. (1974). Intravenous anesthetics: coronary blood flow and myocardial oxygen consumption (with special reference to Althesine). *Acta anaesthesiologica Belgica* **25,** 384—99.
30. Zindler, M. (1976). Etomidate, a new short-acting intravenous hypnotic. Proceedings of the Belgian Congress of Anesthesiology II, Brussels, 10—13 September 1975. *Acta anaesthesiologica Belgica* **27,** 143—52.
31. Vercruysse, P., Hanegreefs, G. and Delooz, H. (1976). Clinical use of etomidate, influence on blood pressure and heart rate. Comparison with thiopentone and methohexital. Proceedings of the Belgian Congress of Anesthesiology II, Brussels, 10—13 September 1975. *Acta anaesthesiologica Belgica* **27,** 153—66.
32. Lamalle, D. (1976). Cardiovascular effects of various anesthetics in man. Four short-acting intravenous anesthetics: Althesin, etomidate, methohexital and propanidid. Proceedings of the Belgian Congress of Anesthesiology II, Brussels, 10—13 September 1975. *Acta anaesthesiologica Belgica* **27,** 208—24.

33. Zindler, M. (1975). Cardiovascular effects of etomidate. In: *Recent Progress in Anaesthesiology and Resuscitation,* Proceedings of the IV European Congress of Anaesthesiology, Madrid, 5—11 September 1974, pp. 118—21. Ed. by A. Arias, R. Llaurado, M. A. Nalda and J. N. Lunn. Excerpta Medica, Amsterdam; American Elsevier, New York.
34. Janssen, P. A. J., Niemegeers, C. J. E. and Marsbook, R. P. H. (1975). Etomidate, a potent non-barbiturate hypnotic. Intravenous etomidate in mice, rats, guinea-pigs, rabbits and dogs. *Archives internationales de pharmacodynamie et de thérapie* **214**, 92—132.
35. Xhonneux, R., Carmeliet, E. and Reneman, R. S. (1975). The electrophysiological effects of etomidate (R-26490), a new, short-acting hypnotic, in various cardiac tissues. In: *Recent Progress in Anaesthesiology and Resuscitation.* Proceedings of the IV European Congress of Anaesthesiology, Madrid, 5—11 September 1974, pp. 157—61. Ed. by A. Arias, R. Llaurado, M. A. Nalda and J. N. Lunn. Excerpta Medica, Amsterdam; American Elsevier, New York.
36. Reneman, R. S., Jageneau, A. H. M., Xhonneux, R. and Laduron, P. (1975). The cardiovascular pharmacology of etomidate (R-26490), a new, potent and short-acting intravenous hypnotic agent. In: *Recent Progress in Anaesthesiology and Resuscitation,* Proceedings of the IV European Congress of Anaesthesiology, Madrid, 5—11 September 1974, pp. 152—6. Ed. by Arias, L. Llaurado, M. A. Nalda and J. N. Lunn. Exceprta Medica, Amsterdam; American Elsevier, New York.
37. Weymar, A., Eigenheer, F., Gethmann, J. W., Reinecke, A., Patschke, D., Tarnow, J. and Bruckner, J. B. (1974). Tierexperimentelle Untersuchungen zur Wirkung von Etomidate auf den Kreislauf und die myokardiale Sauerstoffversorgung. *Anaesthesist* **23,** 150.
38. Bruckner, J. B., Gethmann, J. W., Patschke, D., Tarnow, J. and Weymar, A. (1974). Investigations in the effect of etomidate on the human circulation. *Anaesthesist* **23,** 322—30.
39. Hempelmann, G., Hempelmann, W., Piepenbrock, S., Oster, W. and Karliczek, G. (1974). Blood gas analyses and haemodynamic studies on heart surgery patients using etomidate. *Anaesthesist* **23,** 423—9.
40. Bruckner, J. B. (1976). Etomidate. *Abstract 31,* Sixth World Congress of Anaesthesiology, Mexico City, April 24—30. Excerpta Medica, Amsterdam.
41. van Aken, J. and Rolly, G. (1976). Influence of etomidate, a new short-acting anesthetic agent, on cerebral blood flow in man. Proceedings of the Belgian Congress of Anesthesiology II, Brussels, 10—13 September 1975. *Acta anaesthesiologica Belgica* **27,** 175—80.
42. Lazarevic, Z. D., Rejger, V., Popescu, D. T. and Mattigaly, R. (1976). The influence of hypnomidate on intracranial pressure. *Abstract 235,* sixth World Congress of Anaesthesiology, Mexico City, April 24—30. Excerpta Medica, Amsterdam.

43. Zacharias, M., Dundee, J. W. and Clarke, R. S. J. (1978). Evaluation of etomidate. *British Journal of Anaesthesia* **50,** 633—4.
44. Doenicke, A. (1974). Etomidate, a new intravenous hypnotic. *Acta anaesthesiologica Belgica* **25,** 307—15.
45. Salinas, A. F. (1976). Clinical evaluation of etomidate as an anesthesia-inducing agent. Study of 50 cases. *Abstract 191,* Sixth World Congress of Anaesthesiology, Mexico City, April 24—30. Excerpta Medica, Amsterdam.
46. Kay, B. (1976). A dose-response relationship for etomidate, with some observations on cumulation. *British Journal of Anaesthesia* **48,** 213—16.
47. Clarke, R. S. J. and Dundee, J. W. (1966). Clinical studies of induction agents. XV: A comparison of the cumulative effects of thiopentone, methohexitone and propanidid. *British Journal of Anaesthesia* **38,** 401—5.
48. Dundee, J. W. (1962). Clinical studies of induction agents. III: The relation between duration of anaesthesia and dosage with G 29,505. *British Journal of Anaesthesia* **34,** 790—6.
49. Carson, I. W., Graham, J. and Dundee, J. W. (1975). Clinical studies of induction agents. XLIII: Recovery from Althesin — a comparative study with thiopentone and methohexitone. *British Journal of Anaesthesia* **47,** 358—64.
50. Hannington-Kiff, J. G. (1970). Measurement of recovery from out-patients general anaesthesia with a simple ocular test. *British Medical Journal* **3,** 132—5.
51. Clarke, R. S. J., Dundee, J. W. and Hamilton, R. C. (1967). Interactions between induction agents and muscle relaxants: clinical observations. *Anaesthesia* **22,** 235—48.
52. Hewitt, J. C., Hamilton, R. C., O'Donnell, J. F. and Dundee, J. W. (1966). Clinical studies of induction agents. XIV: A comparative study of venous complications following thiopentone, methohexitone and propanidid. *British Journal of Anaesthesia* **38,** 115—18.
53. O'Donnell, J. F., Hewitt, J. C. and Dundee, J. W. (1969). Clinical studies of induction agents. XXVIII: A further comparison of venous complications following thiopentone, methohexitone and propanidid. *British Journal of Anaesthesia* **41,** 681—3.
54. Carson, I. W., Alexander, J. P., Hewitt, J. C. and Dundee, J. W. (1972). Clinical studies of induction agents: XLI: Venous sequelae following the use of the steroid anaesthetic agent, Althesin. *British Journal of Anaesthesia* **44,** 1311—13.
55. Dundee, J. W. (1978). Total intravenous anaesthesia. *British Journal of Anaesthesia* **50,** 9—10.
56. Tarnow, J., Passian, J., Patschke, D., Weymar, A. and Bruckner, J. P. (1974). Nierendurchblutung unter Etomidate. *Anaesthesist* **23,** 421—2.
57. Editorial (1976). Etomidate. *British Journal of Anaesthesia* **48,** 183.

7

Benzodiazepine sedation — amnesia

The benzodiazepines are not primarily intravenous anaesthetics, though they have been used for this purpose. Rather they are a group of drugs which produce a dose-related degree of cerebral depression. Their effects can vary from tranquillity, sedation or drowsiness to actual anaesthesia. Their main use in anaesthetic practice is for premedication, but they also are of value in the long-term sedation of patients on ventilators and in the production of amnesia in dentistry. These latter two uses depend partly on the ability of the benzodiazepines to produce anterograde amnesia as well as mild sedation.

Of the large number of drugs available, only a few have a place in anaesthesia. Nitrazepam (Mogadon) can be used as a night-time sedation or as preanaesthetic medication, but its actions are not qualitatively different from those of diazepam. Chlordiazepoxide is mainly employed in psychiatric practice. Several other drugs are available only in tablet form while clonazepam, although available in solution, is recommended for use as an anticonvulsant.

Figure 7.1 shows the formulae of the three compounds which are discussed in this chapter: diazepam, flunitrazepam and lorazepam.

Diazepam Flunitrazepam Lorazepam

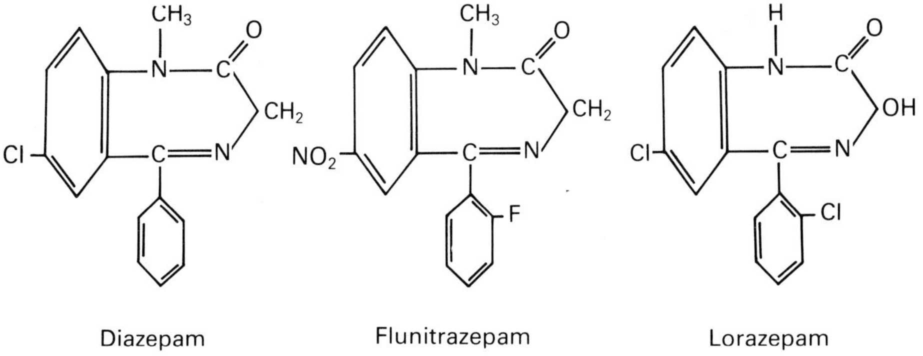

Fig. 7.1 Formulae of diazepam, flunitrazepam and lorazepam.

Diazepam is the 'standard preparation' with which newer members of this group will be compared. It can be given by the oral, intravenous and intramuscular routes, although the latter is too painful and its uptake is too erratic for routine use. Table 7.1 lists its important clinical actions.

Table 7.1 Some important properties of intravenous diazepam

Advantages	Disadvantages
Good tranquillizer in low doses	Not soluble in water
Anti-convulsant	Irritant to veins
Brief amnesic action	Slow onset of action
Atropine not required preoperatively	Variability in response
High safety margin	Prolonged action
Hypersensitivity is rare	

Flunitrazepam (Rohypnol) is a new and more potent drug which has an action very similar to that of diazepam. It has been widely used in continental Europe (Rizzi, Butera and Vendramin, 1975) but is not yet available in Britain.

Lorazepam (Ativan) has been used for a number of years in psychiatric practice and is only recently available in an injectable form. It is more powerful than diazepam but has a slower onset and more prolonged action.

In this chapter the intravenous use of these three drugs as induction agents and for the production of light sedation will be discussed, as will be their relative amnesic actions. Emphasis will be placed on recent data relating to their pharmacology and clinical use. This produces some imbalance in the chapter, but it is assumed that readers are familiar with the basic action of the benzodiazepines.

Induction of anaesthesia

As stated above, the benzodiazepines should not be looked upon as primary induction agents. With diazepam and flunitrazepam there is a delay of 60—90 seconds before the maximum depressant effect occurs; this can be as long as 10—20 minutes with lorazepam, which clearly should never be used as an induction agent. This, however, is not the reason for not recommending the first two drugs as induction agents. Their main disadvantages are their variability in response and their prolonged action.

Individual variability of action is marked with both drugs. For example, Brown and Dundee (1968) found that doses of 0.2 $mg \cdot kg^{-1}$ diazepam produced effects varying from slight drowsiness to onset of sleep. The 'anaesthetic' dose varied from 0.2 to 1.8 $mg \cdot kg^{-1}$ diazepam and from 0.02 to 0.16 $mg \cdot kg^{-1}$ flunitrazepam (Dundee *et al.*, 1976). It is hard to explain this variability but Fig. 7.2 shows great individual variation in plasma levels following 1 $mg \cdot kg^{-1}$ given to six women of similar build and physical status. It does not offer any clues as to the reason for the variations. Perhaps differences in plasma binding are responsible.

This variation also applies, but to a lesser extent, when they are used in smaller doses for mild sedation or for the production of amnesia.

Although patients seem to recover quickly from the effects of small doses of diazepam, this can be deceptive. High plasma levels persist for up to 24

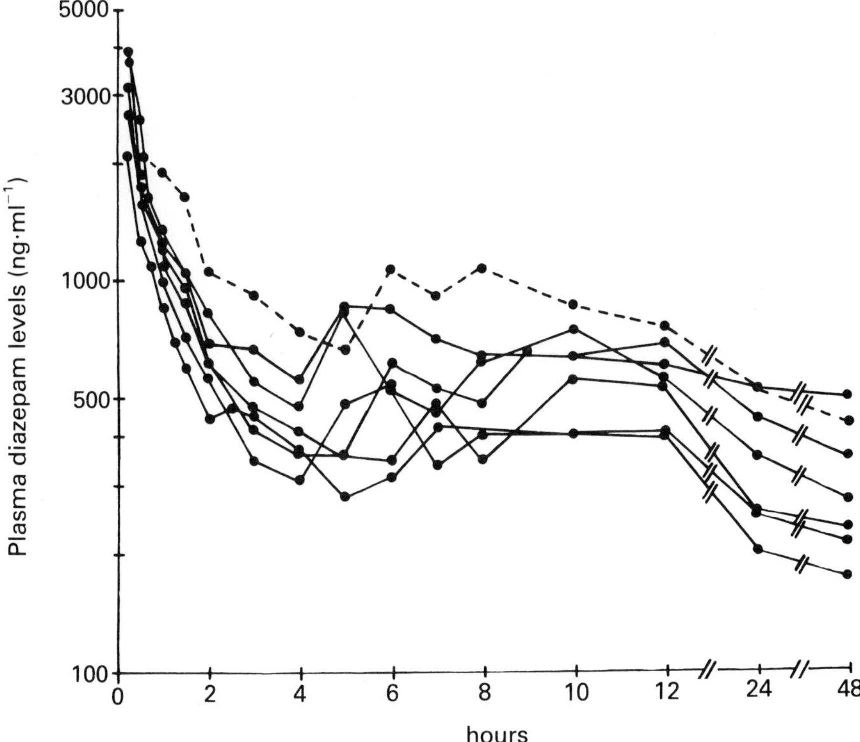

Fig. 7.2 Plasma diazepam levels in 7 patients following 1 mg·kg^{-1} intravenously. Levels indicated by the dashed line occurred in a patient who was significantly lighter than others.

hours after the single oral or intramuscular administration of 10 mg to adults (Gamble, Dundee and Assaf, 1975). This is to be expected in view of the half-life of 93.2 hours found by Mahon *et al.* (1976) following the initial distribution phase. There is no reason to believe that the drug will be eliminated more rapidly if given intravenously (Baird and Hailey, 1972; Gamble, Mackay and Dundee, 1973).

The main metabolite of diazepam, *N*-desmethyl diazepam, is only slightly less potent than the parent compound as a sedative and muscle relaxant in animals (Randall, Scheckel and Banziger, 1965). In view of the delayed recovery which sometimes occurs with large doses it is probable that this also applies in man. The average plasma levels of diazepam and *N*-desmethyl diazepam found in ten subjects after 1 mg·kg^{-1} intravenously (Fig. 7.3) show a number of interesting features. There is a steady increase in *N*-desmethyl diazepam levels over the first 24 hours and thereafter the concentration of metabolite declines at approximately the same rate as that of diazepam. This must cause prolonged drowsiness. One also notes an increase in plasma diazepam levels 6—8 hours after its administration, with a second smaller increase at around 10—12 hours. This is thought to be due to enterohepatic

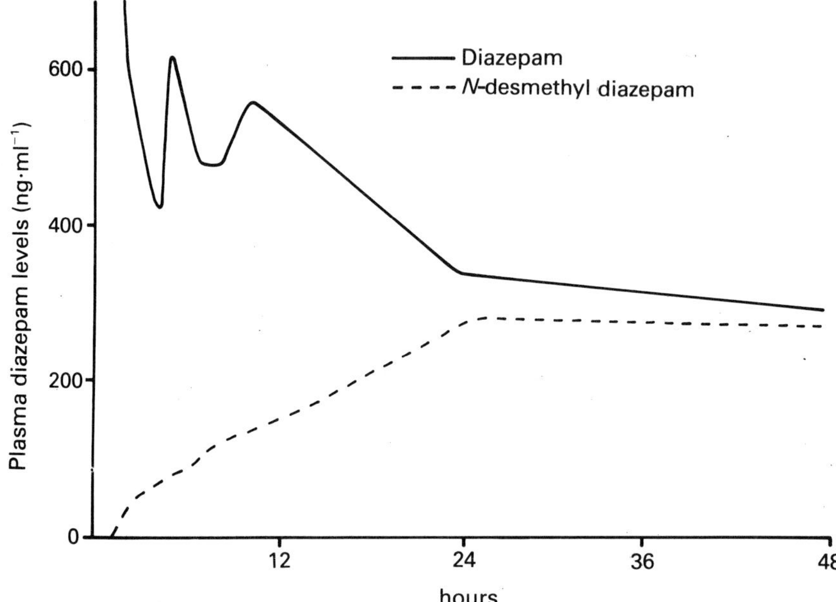

Fig. 7.3 Average plasma levels of diazepam and *N*-desmethyl diazepam in 10 patients following 1 mg·kg^{-1} intravenously.

recirculation (Van der Kleijn *et al.*, 1971; Korttila, Mattila and Linnoila, 1976), although Mahon and his colleagues (1976) were unable to detect diazepam or *N*-desmethyl diazepam in human bile.

Irrespective of its causation, the rise in plasma levels which occurs around the 6–8 hour period after injection is of clinical importance because patients may have a tendency to fall asleep again at this time. When smaller doses of diazepam are given for outpatient dentistry in the morning and patients allowed to go home (apparently fully recovered), they may drop off to sleep again around 16.00–18.00 hours. If they happen to be in heavy traffic or close to machinery at this time, then this could be dangerous.

Diazepam is metabolized primarily in the liver. Andreasen and his colleagues (1976) from Copenhagen have compared its elimination in patients with hepatic cirrhosis and in normal subjects. Although the dose used was small (10 mg), they showed a fivefold increase in the terminal half-life from 32 hours in the absence of liver damage to 164 hours in cirrhotic patients, although the rapid initial disposition rate constant was similar in both groups. Brown (1977) has suggested that a reduction in hepatic blood flow, by diminishing the availability of the drug to the biotransformation enzymes located in the endoplasmic reticulum of the hepatic cell, may play a part in this delayed clearance. There is clear evidence that the cirrhotic patient maintains a relatively high concentration of diazepam in the circulation for a longer time than does the normal patient. While this is important in any circumstances, it is especially important when large induction doses are given. Klotz *et al.* (1975) had previously demonstrated an increase in half-life of flunitrazepam with increasing age of the patient, which was interpreted as being due to decreased metabolism.

One has no reason to believe that the cardiovascular effects of large doses of diazepam will be less than those of orthodox anaesthetics. There is a widely held view that small doses are less likely to cause hypotension than barbiturates but Lyons, Clarke and Dundee (1974) were unable to confirm this in a study carried out in patients scheduled for cardiac surgery. Comparable doses of all induction agents appeared to produce a similar fall in blood pressure but, whereas the fall occurred within 1 minute with thiopentone, there was a delay of 2–3 minutes with diazepam. If laryngoscopy is carried out during this time then the maximum depressant effects of the benzodiazepines will be antagonized.

Clarke and Lyons (1977) have shown the similarity between the cardiovascular effects of equivalent doses of diazepam and lorazepam in patients having cardiac operations. Figure 7.4 shows the average changes in heart rate with the two benzodiazepines and suggests that they may be preferable to thiopentone in this respect. These authors also studied diazepam at three dose levels (0.21, 0.46 and 0.60 mg·kg^{-1}) and concluded that 'if a smooth induction is considered important, the risks of giving diazepam 0.6 mg·kg^{-1} are no greater than with 0.2 mg·kg^{-1})'.

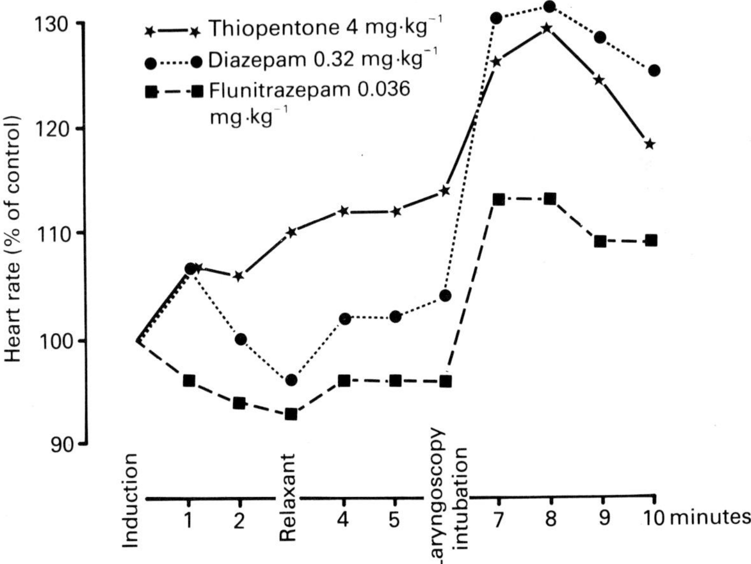

Fig. 7.4 Average changes in heart rate, expressed as percentage of the control value during induction of anaesthesia in three groups, each of 20 patients given thiopentone 4 mg·kg^{-1}, diazepam 0.32 mg·kg^{-1} and flunitrazepam 0.036 mg·kg^{-1}. (From Clarke and Lyons, 1977.)

Despite earlier views to the contrary (Steen *et al.*, 1966; Zsigmond and Shiveley, 1966), there is little doubt that even small doses of diazepam affect the respiration. Catchlove and Kafer (1971) found that a dose of 0.14 $mg{\cdot}kg^{-1}$ produced significant increases in V_D/V_T and Pa_{CO_2} and a decrease in V_T. It depresses the ventilatory response to CO_2 and modifies the characteristics of gas exchange within the lung. These changes are of no significance in normal patients (Gasser and Bellville, 1976) but may be important with large doses such as are used for the intravenous induction of anaesthesia, or in patients with respiratory impairment (Lakshminarayan *et al.*, 1976). During anaesthesia, where spontaneous ventilation is permitted, diazepam anaesthesia should be accompanied by an increased inspired oxygen concentration.

Another possible side effect of the use of larger doses of the drugs is an impairment of liver function but Clarke *et al.* (1974) found no evidence of this in patients given 0.62—0.65 $mg{\cdot}kg^{-1}$ diazepam. Its effect on the diseased liver is not known but it does not appear to affect kidney function and may be given to patients undergoing renal clearance studies or those with a pre-existing renal insufficiency (Guignard *et al.*, 1975).

Mild sedation

All three intravenous benzodiazepines are capable of producing mild sedation in small doses. This is useful for patients undergoing operations under local anaesthesia, including endoscopy. With spinal or epidural anaesthesia patients who are not sedated may get restless, whereas with a small dose of diazepam they will often fall asleep during the operation. Similarly, intravenous diazepam has made conservative dentistry under local anaesthesia acceptable to many patients who would otherwise insist on general anaesthesia.

Theoretically the anti-convulsant action of the benzodiazepines may be of value in patients having local anaesthesia (Wesseling, 1973) but the clinical importance of this is not known.

One must remember that benzodiazepines are not analgesics. They will not make up for poor regional techniques or for an inadequate spinal or extradural block. Although, strictly speaking, they do not enhance the action of narcotic analgesics, in practice the reduction of anxiety and the soporific action make the combination useful. Combinations such as diazepam—pentazocine, which can be used for endoscopy, are discussed in Chapter 9.

In most circumstances diazepam is the drug of choice for mild sedation, although preliminary observations suggest that, in appropriate doses, flunitrazepam has an action which is indistinguishable from that of diazepam. Both produce their maximum effect in 60—90 seconds but the clinical effect of flunitrazepam may persist slightly longer. Either of these can be given as ‘instant premedication’ and they will quickly allay the apprehension of most patients. In contrast, the slower onset of lorazepam necessitates its early administration. Its use in more prolonged procedures is worth exploring.

In certain circumstances the amnesic action of the benzodiazepines plays a major part in their clinical usefulness as mild sedatives. This will now be discussed in detail.

Amnesia

The ability of diazepam, flunitrazepam and lorazepam to partially or completely obtund recall of events following their intravenous injection is well established. This action is infrequent when normal premedicant and sedative doses are given by mouth or by intramuscular injection. None of the benzodiazepines causes any retrograde amnesia.

Following the injection of 10 mg diazepam intravenously the peak amnesic action occurs in about 2 minutes and persists for approximately 5 minutes; thereafter it declines over the next 30—40 minutes (Dundee and Pandit, 1972). Figure 7.5 summarizes the findings of a comparative study in which George and Dundee (1977) evaluated the ability of patients to recall objects shown to them following comparable doses of the three benzodiazepines.

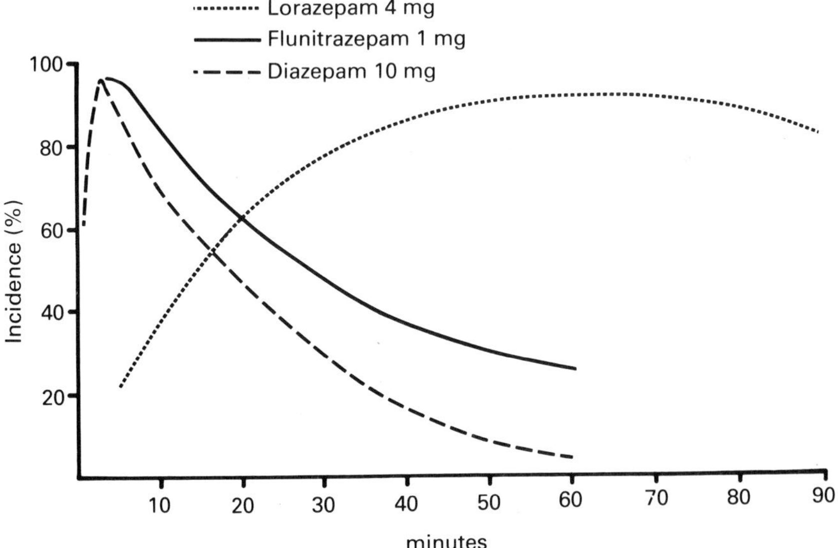

Fig. 7.5 Percentage incidence of patients who could not recall being shown objects at various times following the intravenous administration of diazepam 10 mg, flunitrazepam 1 mg and lorazepam 4 mg. (From George and Dundee, 1977.)

This shows the slower onset and longer amnesic action of lorazepam, as compared with the other two drugs. Heisterkamp and Cohen (1975) have shown that impairment of memory may persist for up to 6 hours after lorazepam.

The amnesic action of any of the benzodiazepines is most marked when they produce sedation. Patients may doze off to sleep but can be readily roused. Even if they are shown an object which they can recognize or are spoken to and respond sensibly, recall for these events will be suppressed. The medicolegal implications of this are fairly obvious. If one attempts to prolong the amnesic action of diazepam by increasing the dose, the soporific effect will become more marked (Fig. 7.6).

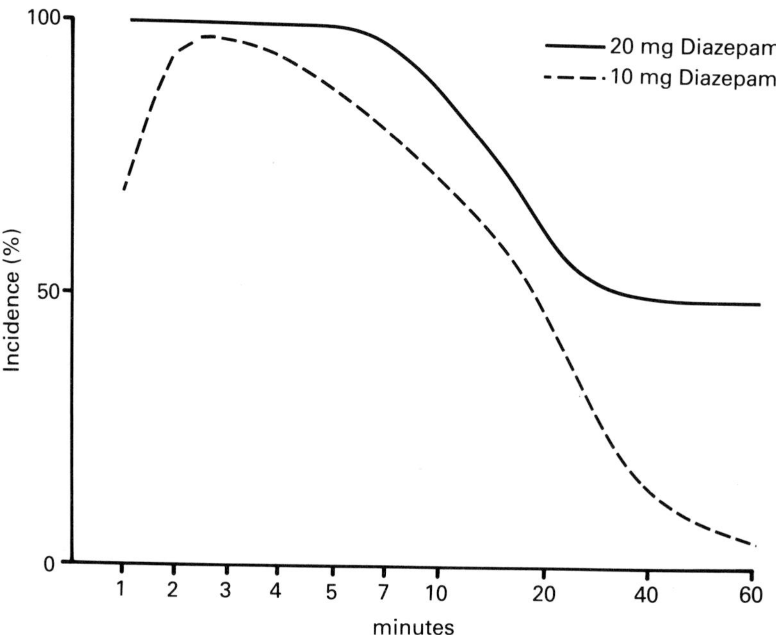

Fig. 7.6 Comparison of the incidence of amnesia after 10 and 20 mg diazepam.

Obstetrics

In order to minimize the pharmacological effects of drugs on the mother and fetus, very light anaesthesia is used for operative obstetric procedures. There are a great many reports of patients who are not fully anaesthetized and who recall events during the operation. In 1969 Wilson and Turner reported that, of patients anaesthetized for caesarean section with thiopentone, nitrous oxide and a neuromuscular blocking drug, 8—9 per cent had undoubted factual recall of events which had occurred during anaesthesia.

This was not lessened by premedication with diazepam (Turner and Wilson, 1969). More recently, Ng and Gurubatham (1974) found a 25 per cent incidence of recall of unpleasant nature in primigravidi of 30 years or older; Chakraborty, Chakraborty and Pandit (1974) found that 5 out of 139 patients undergoing caesarean section clearly recalled events during surgery, while Stovner and Vangen (1974) found recall in between 12 and 35 per cent of patients, depending on the anaesthetic used. These reports from three different countries show the extent of the problem and in this field the amnesic action of the benzodiazepines could be of value. To use this to its best advantage one has to appreciate the dose-response effect of the different drugs and, in particular, how these vary in relation to the route of administration and also the expected duration of amnesia.

From the data previously presented it would seem unlikely that premedication with 10—15 mg diazepam will affect the incidence of recall during operation. Diazepam does not cause retrograde amnesia and its intravenous administration when the baby is delivered will not affect recall of events prior to this. A small dose given 5—10 minutes prior to delivery will certainly contribute to amnesia but its placental transmission and potential effects on the fetus have to be considered. There would seem to be safer methods to prevent recall.

A number of workers have shown that diazepam rapidly crosses into the placenta (Cavanagh and Condo, 1964; Owen, Irani and Blair, 1972; Cree, Meyer and Hailey, 1973). Scher, Hailey and Beard (1972) and Yeh *et al.* (1974) found that maximum plasma diazepam levels were recorded 5—10 minutes after its administration to the mother, although Gamble *et al.* (1977) found that the ratio of cord and maternal plasma concentrations did not reach their maximum until about 1 hour after injection.

Dawes (1973) has suggested that distribution of a drug in the mother causes a rapid fall in maternal plasma levels and that fetal levels of a drug which rapidly crosses the placental barrier may be higher than the maternal levels until a steady state is reached. This may explain why Erkkola, Kanto and Sellman (1974) found that diazepam levels in infants were higher than the mothers' following a single administration whereas the ratio was reversed in mothers on long-term diazepam therapy.

Gamble and his colleagues (1977) found that plasma levels in the mother decline at similar rates to those in the fetus during the first 24 hours after delivery, as shown in Table 7.2.

Table 7.2 Average plasma levels of diazepam found in the mother and fetus following 10 mg given intravenously to the mother

	Mean plasma diazepam ($ng \cdot ml^{-1}$)	
	Delivery	24 hours
Mother	134 ± 17.6	46 ± 1.2
Infant	196 ± 21.1	75 ± 8.4
P	<0.001	<0.001

The anti-convulsant action of diazepam has led to its use in the treatment of pre-eclampsia. One regimen of therapy consisted of the intravenous injection of 10—20 mg followed by the slow administration of 40 mg diluted in 500 ml aqueous solution of dextrose. In view of the data on the placental transmission of the benzodiazepines, one is not surprised that many babies were born with evidence of diazepam overdose, hypotonia and hypothermia being the most common complications. These complications should not lead to the abandonment of diazepam but rather its dosage should be restricted and it should be combined with other anti-convulsants such as chlormethiazole or with an extradural block.

A limited study of the placental transmission of lorazepam has been carried out by McBride and his colleagues (1979). With this drug fetal levels do not exceed those in the mother (Fig. 7.7) and the neonate can dispose of the drug at the same rate as the mother. In practice the intravenous injection of 2.5 mg lorazepam early in the first stage of labour or even prior to rupture of the amniotic membranes produced excellent sedation; mothers relaxed and slept between pains and the patients appeared to require smaller doses of analgesics.

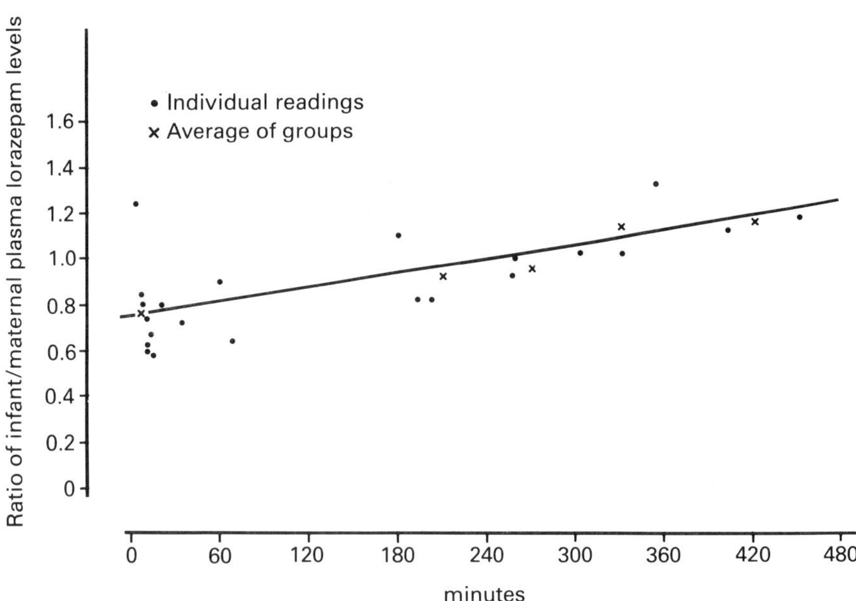

Fig. 7.7 Ratio of infant to maternal plasma lorazepam, at different times following intravenous administration of 2.5 mg to the mother. In some patients the drug was given prior to induction of labour and in others during the second stage. (McBride *et al.*, 1979.)

Long-term sedation

Diazepam and lorazepam have been used to produce sedation and amnesia in patients on long-term treatment in intensive therapy units (Dundee, Johnston and Gray, 1976). Diazepam is the more 'flexible' of the two drugs; after the first two doses it produces a long period of sedation and can be given at 4-hourly intervals. There is some delay in the onset of action of lorazepam but it has proved free from side effects, even after very large total doses of up to 500 mg.

A cumulation of diazepam and its metabolite might be anticipated after prolonged use, resulting in a delay in recovery. Figure 7.8 is typical of the plasma concentration of diazepam and *N*-desmethyl diazepam found following 10 mg diazepam 4-hourly for 18 days. A similar fall in plasma concentration has been found with lorazepam, but in this case there was no major metabolite which could contribute to its hypnotic action. Despite these high plasma levels, clinical recovery was not prolonged. This suggests that a considerable degree of cerebral tolerance occurs to the depressant effects of the benzodiazepines.

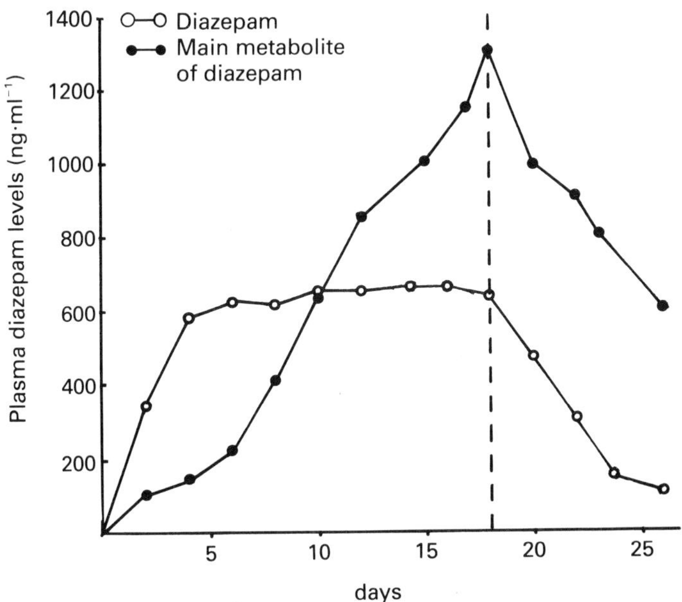

Fig. 7.8 Typical plasma levels of diazepam and its main metabolite following the intravenous administration of 10 mg 4-hourly for 18 days. The vertical dashed line shows when the therapy was stopped. (From Gamble, Dundee and Gray, 1976.)

Dentistry

Reference has been made in Chapter 4 to the use of diazepam prior to conservative dentistry. The brief period of amnesia which follows 10—15 mg in adults not only 'settles' the patients at the beginning of the procedure, but produces amnesia for the injection of the local anaesthetic. In equivalent doses, flunitrazepam has a slightly longer amnesic action which could be advantageous.

It should be remembered that diazepam is not free from cardiovascular effects; Jenkinson and his colleagues (1974) found a significant fall in cardiac output and stroke volume, with increase in heart rate and peripheral resistance when doses of 12.5—17.5 mg were used as a sedative for oral surgery. However, in the light of other reports (Healy, Robinson and Vickers, 1970), one has to weigh these against the effects of fear on the haemodynamics of poor-risk cardiac patients.

Table 4.3 shows the delay in recovery following diazepam, as compared with Althesin, but, even taking this into consideration, the benzodiazepines would appear to be the safer drugs. If flunitrazepam should become commercially available for intravenous use, it is likely to be preferred to either of the other compounds.

Electrical cardioversion

The mild sedative and amnesic action of diazepam has recommended its use prior to direct current cardioversion (Nutter and Massumi, 1965). It enjoys considerable popularity in this field, not only because of its unique sedative properties but also because it obviates the need for an anaesthetist (Glassman, 1971; Somers *et al.*, 1971).

Muenster and his colleagues (1967) reported the occurrence of ventricular extrasystoles in 11 of 18 patients induced with thiopentone prior to cardioversion but in none of 19 patients anaesthetized with diazepam. The most complete comparison of different agents in cardioversion is reported by Orko (1976) from Helsinki who anaesthetized three groups of 50 patients with diazepam or thiopentone or propanidid. An average dose of 4.6 $mg \cdot kg^{-1}$ propanidid resulted in more hypotension than diazepam (0.32 $mg \cdot kg^{-1}$) or thiopentone (3.7 $mg \cdot kg^{-1}$). Apnoea was most frequent following thiopentone and spontaneous involuntary muscle movements were most prominent after propanidid. Successful conversion of dysrhythmia occurred more frequently when diazepam was used (84 per cent), than with thiopentone (72 per cent) or propanidid (70 per cent), although these differences are not significantly different. However, one-third of those receiving diazepam recalled the cardioversion, an incidence which was unacceptably high. Thiopentone was both pleasant and suitable for cardioversion but diazepam is especially recommended for poor-risk patients and in emergency situations.

Miscellaneous uses

Among the various fields in which the clinical anaesthetist may find a use for intravenous diazepam is the treatment of severe delirium tremens

(Thompson *et al.*, 1975). An initial dose of 10 mg is followed by 5 mg every 4 minutes until a calm state occurs and this is then followed by 5—10 mg given every 1-4 hours as required. This technique is preferable to the use of paraldehyde.

The amnesic and sedative effects of diazepam commend its use in patients undergoing cardiac catheterization. Healy (1969) has reported on the excellent conditions which it affords, with minimal effects on ventilation. Markiewicz and his colleagues (1976) from Stanford have studied the circulatory effects of 10 mg in their patients. Following the diazepam the heart rate rose considerably, accompanied by a significant fall in aortic, systolic and left ventricular pressures. Although the average changes were minor they were clinically significant in some individual patients. Anxiolysis and sedation were excellent. These authors caution lest the data obtained from cardiac catheterization are taken to reflect the action of the diazepam in healthy patients. Nevertheless, they recommend that its use in patients with coronary artery disease be further investigated.

Venous sequelae

Opinions vary about the incidence and severity of venous sequelae after the injection of the benzodiazepines. Hegarty and Dundee (1977) have reported a study in which patients were given roughly equivalent doses of undiluted preparations of diazepam, lorazepam, flunitrazepam and then followed up for 10 days. The findings are considered to be of such great clinical importance that they are discussed here at length. Table 7.3 shows that at 7—10 days after injection there was a significantly higher incidence of venous sequelae among patients who had received diazepam than among those who had received lorazepam ($P<0.02$) or flunitrazepam ($P<0.0005$).

Table 7.3 Incidence of sequelae occurring 2—3 days and 7—10 days after the intravenous injection of three benzodiazepines (Hegarty and Dundee, 1977)

Drug	Dose (mg)	No.	Total venous sequelae (%)	
			2—3 days	7—10 days
Diazepam	10	44	23	39
Lorazepam	4	40	8	15
Flunitrazepam	1—2	43	0	5

The incidence with these latter two drugs did not differ significantly. Both thrombosis (7 per cent) and phlebitis (5 per cent) were found on the second or third days after diazepam, but not with the other two benzodiazepines. Painless thrombosis was the only complication noted at 7—10 days, by which time it had often extended to the upper arm and even into the axilla. In a few patients in whom it was possible to continue observations, thrombosis was found to persist for several weeks. Very long thrombosed segments of vein were found more often after diazepam. A few patients in this study received more than one drug and Table 7.4 demonstrates that diazepam is worse than the other two drugs in respect of its action on the veins.

Table 7.4 Occurrence of venous thrombosis (+) on 7th—10th day in patients receiving more than one benzodiazepine on separate occasions

	Diazepam	Lorazepam	Flunitrazepam
M, 76	+		—
F, 70	+	—	—
M, 34	—	+	—
M, 28	—	—	
M, 44	—		—
M, 49	+	—	
M, 18	—		—
M, 62		—	—
M, 39	—	—	

Table 7.5 analyses the effect of a number of factors on the incidence of painless thrombosis and, as expected, this occurs most frequently when small hand or wrist vessels are used for injection. Of equal clinical importance is the age of the patient. Figure 7.9 is drawn from the data of Hegarty and Dundee and pertains only to diazepam. The incidence of thrombosis is unacceptably high in elderly patients.

Table 7.5 Some factors influencing the incidence of painless venous thrombosis found in 7—10 days after intravenous injection of benzodiazepines

Size of vein		Location		Combination	
Large	13%	Antecubital	12%	Large antecubital	6%
Small and moderate	26%	Wrist and hand	24%	Small hand or wrist	23%
Difference	NS		NS		$P<0.05$

NS = not significant

A much lower incidence of venous thrombosis is one of the positive advantages of flunitrazepam over diazepam. At the time of writing (March 1978), flunitrazepam is not available commercially. Should it be introduced into clinical practice this lower incidence alone would be sufficient to commend it over diazepam. The reports quoted here relate to undiluted lorazepam (4 mg·ml^{-1}); the manufacturers now recommend that this should be diluted with an equal volume of saline in order to reduce its irritant effect to a level comparable with flunitrazepam.

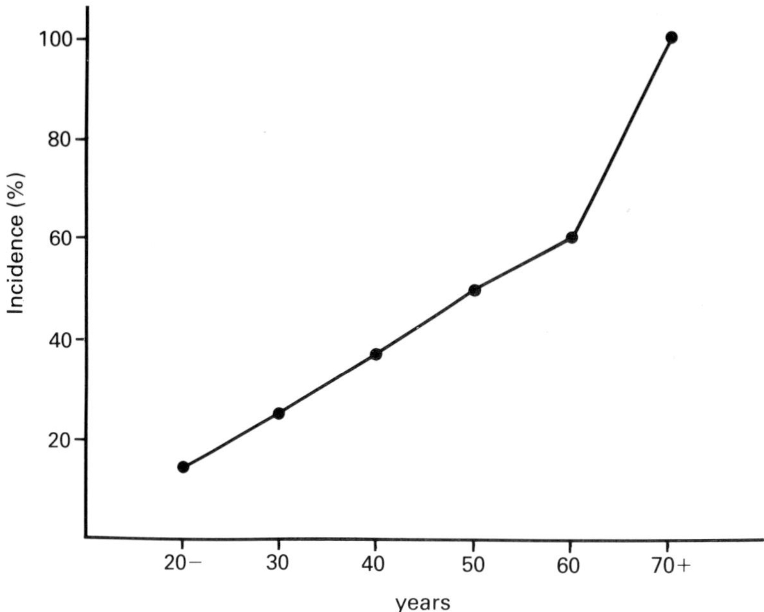

Fig. 7.9 Percentage incidence of thrombosis, found 7—10 days after intravenous injection of 10 mg diazepam, related to the age of the patients.

Physostigmine reversal

Physostigmine, being a tertiary amine, crosses the blood-brain barrier and increases brain acetylcholine concentration by inhibition of cholinesterase. It has been used successfully in ameliorating the 'central cholinergic syndrome' which may be induced by atropine, hyoscine, tricyclic antidepressants and anti-parkinson drugs (Holzgrafe, Vondrell and Mintz, 1973). There is increasing clinical evidence that it can reverse central depression induced by benzodiazepine tranquillizers.

Little is known about the specificity of this action but there are several reports which show that physostigmine may act as an antidote to an occasional marked depressant effect of diazepam (Larson, Hurlbert and Wingard, 1977). It has also proved effective in overdose in a child (DiLiberti, O'Brien and Turner, 1975). Although untoward effects from diazepam, such as respiratory arrest, are uncommon and are best treated with ventilation, it is useful to have physostigmine available. The adult dose is 1—2 mg given slowly and repeated as required.

Delirium following lorazepam has also been treated successfully with physostigmine (Blitt and Petty, 1975).

Where next?

The benzodiazepines are well established as minor tranquillizers (Garattini, Mussini and Randall, 1973). Some of their depressant actions are of use in anaesthesia and these have been discussed. With the advent of lorazepam we now have available both long- and short-acting drugs with a very similar quality of action (Table 7.6). We certainly do not need both diazepam and flunitrazepam. Diazepam is so well established in clinical practice that one wonders whether the advantages of flunitrazepam are sufficient to justify its commercial introduction. Having personally followed up patients with extended venous thrombosis after diazepam, the author has no doubt that flunitrazepam is a superior agent. One hopes that commercial interests and restrictive drug regulations will not prevent its advantages being passed on to the public. With flunitrazepam and lorazepam we have an excellent range of benzodiazepine activity. All that is now required is a water-soluble preparation.

Table 7.6 Summary of the important differences between the three benzodiazepines

	Diazepam	Flunitrazepam	Lorazepam
Equivalent dose (mg)	10	0.5—1.0	2.5—4.0
Onset i.v. (min)	1—2	1—2	5—15
Duration of sedation (above dose)	40—60 min	60—90 min	4—6 h
Proven amnesic action	+	+	+
Has been used for induction of anaesthesia	+ +	+	—
Venous sequelae	+ + +	±	+

References

Andreasen, P. B., Hendel, J., Greisen, G. and Hvidberg, E. F. (1976). Pharmacokinetics of diazepam in disordered liver function. *European Journal of Clinical Pharmacology* **10,** 115—20.

Baird, E. S. and Hailey, D. M. (1972). Delayed recovery from a sedative: correlation of the plasma levels of diazepam with clinical effects after oral and intravenous administration. *British Journal of Anaesthesia* **44,** 803—8.

Blitt, C. D. and Petty, W. C. (1975). Reversal of lorazepam delirium by physostigmine. *Anesthesia and Analgesia . . . Current Researches* **54,** 607—8.

Brown, B. R. (1977). Critique on Andreasen, P. B., Hendel, J., Greisen, G. and Hvidberg, E. F. (1976). European Journal of Clinical Pharmacology, 10, 115—120. *Survey of Anesthesiology* **21,** 225—6.

Brown, S. S. and Dundee, J. W. (1968). Clinical studies of induction agents. XXV: Diazepam. *British Journal of Anaesthesia* **40,** 108—12.

Catchlove, R. F. H. and Kafer, E. R. (1971). The effects of diazepam on the ventilatory response to carbon dioxide and on steady-state gas exchange. *Anesthesiology* **34,** 9—13.

Cavanagh, D. and Condo, C. S. (1964). Diazepam — a pilot study of drug concentrations in maternal blood, amniotic fluid and cord blood. *Current Therapeutic Research* **6,** 122—6.

Chakraborty, S., Chakraborty, R. K. and Pandit, S. K. (1974). Awareness during caesarean section under general anaesthesia: influence of various premedicants. *Indian Journal of Anaesthesia* **22,** 9—13.

Clarke, R. S. J., Dundee, J. W., Doggart, J. R. and Lavery, T. (1974). The effects of single and intermittent administrations of Althesin and other intravenous anesthetic agents on liver function. *Anesthesia and Analgesia . . . Current Researches* **53,** 461—8.

Clarke, R. S. J. and Lyons, S. M. (1977). Diazepam and flunitrazepam as induction agents for cardiac surgical operations. *Acta anaesthesiologica Scandinavica* **21,** 282—92.

Cree, J. E., Meyer, J. and Hailey, D. M. (1973). Diazepam in labour: its metabolism and effect on the clinical condition and thermogenesis of the newborn. *British Medical Journal* **3,** 251—5.

Dawes, G. S. (1973). The distribution and action of drugs on the foetus in utero. *British Journal of Anaesthesia* **45,** 766.

DiLiberti, J., O'Brien, M. L. and Turner, T. (1975). The use of physostigmine as an antidote in accidental diazepam intoxication. *Journal of Pediatrics* **86,** 106—7.

Dundee, J. W., Johnston, H. M. L. and Gray, R. C. (1976). Lorazepam as a sedative—amnesic in an intensive care unit. *Current Medical Research and Opinion* **4,** 290—5.

Dundee, J. W. and Pandit, S. K. (1972). Studies on drug-induced amnesia with intravenous anaesthetic agents in man. *British Journal of Clinical Practice* **26,** 164—6.

Dundee, J. W., Varadarajan, C. R., Gaston, J. H. and Clarke, R. S. J. (1976). Clinical studies of induction agents. XLIII: Flunitrazepam. *British Journal of Anaesthesia* **48,** 551—5.

Erkkola, R., Kanto, J. and Sellman, R. (1974). Diazepam in early human pregnancy. *Acta obstetricia et gynecologica Scandinavica* **53,** 135—8.

Gamble, J. A. S., Dundee, J. W. and Assaf, R. A. E. (1975). Plasma diazepam levels after single dose oral and intramuscular administration. *Anaesthesia* **30,** 164—9.

Gamble, J. A. S., Dundee, J. W. and Gray, R. C. (1976). Plasma diazepam concentrations following prolonged administration. *British Journal of Anaesthesia 48,* 1087—90.

Gamble, J. A. S., Mackay, J. S. and Dundee, J. W. (1973). Plasma levels of diazepam. *British Journal of Anaesthesia* **45,** 1085.

Gamble, J. A. S., Moore, J., Lamki, H. and Howard, P. J. (1977). A study of plasma diazepam levels in mother and infant. *Journal of Obstetrics anbd Gynaecology of the British Commonwealth* **84,** 588—91.

Garattini, S., Mussini, E. and Randall, L. O. (Eds) (1973). *The Benzodiazepines.* Raven Press, New York.

Gasser, J. C. and Bellville, J. W. (1976). The respiratory effects of hydroxyzine, diazepam and pentazocine in man. *Anaesthesia* **31,** 718—23.

George, K. A. and Dundee, J. W. (1977). Relative amnesic actions of diazepam, flunitrazepam and lorazepam in man. *British Journal of Clinical Pharmacology* **4,** 45—50.

Glassman, E. (1971). Direct current cardioversion. *American Heart Journal* **82,** 128.

Guignard, J. P., Filloux, B., Lavoie, J., Pelet, J. and Torrado, A. (1975). Effect of intravenous diazepam on renal function. *Clinical Pharmacology and Therapeutics* **18,** 401—4.

Healy, T. E. J. (1969). Intravenous diazepam for cardiac catheterisation. *Anaesthesia* **24,** 537—40.

Healy, T. E. J., Robinson, J. S. and Vickers, M. D. (1970). Physiological responses to intravenous diazepam as a sedative for conservative dentistry. *British Medical Journal* **3,** 10—13.

Hegarty, J. E. and Dundee, J. W. (1977). Sequelae after the intravenous injection of three benzodiazepines — diazepam, lorazepam and flunitrazepam. *British Medical Journal* **2,** 1384—5.

Heisterkamp, D. V. and Cohen, P. T. (1975). The effect of intravenous premedication with lorazepam (Ativan), pentobarbital and diazepam on recall. *British Journal of Anaesthesia* **47,** 79—81.

Holzgrafe, R. E., Vondrell, J. J. and Mintz, S. M. (1973). Reversal of postoperative reactions to scopolamine with physostigmine. *Anesthesia and Analgesia . . . Current Researches* **52,** 921—5.

Jenkinson, J. L., MacRae, W. R., Scott, D. B. and Gould, J. F. (1974). Haemodynamic effects of diazepam used as a sedative for oral surgery. *British Journal of Anaesthesia* **46,** 294.

Klotz, U., Avant, G. R., Hoyumpa, A., Schenker, S. and Wilkinson, G. R. (1975). The effects of age and liver disease on the disposition and elimination of diazepam in adult man. *Journal of Clinical Investigation* **55,** 347—59.

Korttila, K., Mattila, M. J. and Linnoila, M. (1976). Prolonged recovery after diazepam sedation: the influence of food, charcoal ingestion and injection rate on the effects of intravenous diazepam. *British Journal of Anaesthesia* **48,** 333—40.

Lakshminarayan, S., Sahn, S. A., Hudson, L. E. and Weil, J. V. (1976). Effect of diazepam on ventilatory responses. *Clinical Pharmacology and Therapeutics* **20,** 178—83.

Larson, G. F., Hurlbert, B. J. and Wingard, D. W. (1977). Physostigmine reversal of diazepam-induced depression. *Anesthesia and Analgesia . . . Current Researches* **56,** 348—51.

Lyons, S. M., Clarke, R. S. J. and Dundee, J. W. (1974). Some cardiovascular and respiratory effects of four non-barbiturate anaesthetic induction agents. *European Journal of Clinical Pharmacology* **7,** 275—9.

McBride, R. J., Dundee, J. W., Moore, J., Toner, W. and Howard, P. J. (1979). Placental transfer of lorazepam: Paper read to British Pharmacological Society. January meeting, London.

Mahon, W. A., Inaba, T., Umeda, T., Tsutsumi, E. and Stone, R. (1976). Biliary elimination of diazepam in man. *Clinical Pharmacology and Therapeutics* **19,** 443—50.

Markiewicz, W., Hunt, S., Harrison, D. C. and Alterman, E. L. (1976). Circulatory effects of diazepam in heart disease. *Journal of Clinical Pharmacology* **16,** 637—44.

Muenster, J. J., Rosenberg, M. S., Carleton, R. A. and Graettinger, J. S. (1967). Comparison between diazepam and sodium pentothal during direct current countershock. *Journal of the American Medical Association* **199,** 758.

Ng, K. H. and Gurubatham, A. I. (1974). Awareness during caesarean section under general anaesthesia. *Medical Journal of Australia* **2,** 774—6.

Nutter, D. O. and Massumi, R. A. (1965). Diazepam in cardioversion. *New England Journal of Medicine* **273,** 650.

Orko, R. (1976). Anaesthesia for cardioversion: a comparison of diazepam, thiopentone and propanidid. *British Journal of Anaesthesia* **48,** 257—62.

Owen, J. R., Irani, S. F. and Blair, A. W. (1972). Effect of diazepam administered to mothers during labour on temperature regulation of neonates. *Archives of Disease in Childhood* **47,** 107—10.

Randall, L. O., Scheckel, C. L. and Banziger, R. F. (1965). Pharmacology of the metabolites of chlordiazepoxide and diazepam. *Current Therapeutic Research* **7,** 590—606.

Rizzi, R., Butera, G. and Vendramin, M. L. (1975). Flunitrazepam (Rohypnol) as the only hypnotic agent during general anaesthesia. In: *Recent Progress in Anaesthesiology and Resuscitation.* Proceedings of the IV European Congress of Anaesthesiology, Madrid, 5—11 September 1974, pp. 122—31. Ed. by A. Arias, R. Llaurado, M. A. Nalda and J. N. Lunn. Excerpta Medica, Amsterdam; American Elsevier, New York.

Scher, J., Hailey, D. M. and Beard, R. W. (1972). The effects of diazepam on the foetus. *Journal of Obstetrics and Gynaecology of the British Commonwealth* **79,** 635—8.

Somers, K., Gunstone, R. F., Patel, A. K. and D'Arbela, P. G. (1971). Intravenous diazepam for direct-current cardioversion. *British Medical Journal* **4,** 13.

Steen, S. N., Weitzner, S. W., Amaha, K. and Martinez, L. R. (1966). The effect of diazepam on the respiratory response to carbon dioxide. *Canadian Anaesthetists' Society Journal* **13,** 374—7.

Stovner, J. and Vangen, O. (1974). Diazepam compared to thiopentone as induction agent for caesarean sections. *Acta anaesthesiologica Scandinavica* **18,** 264—9.

Thompson, W. L., Johnson, A. D., Maddrey, W. L. and Osler Medical Housestaff (1975). Diazepam and paraldehyde for the treatment of severe delirium tremens: a controlled trial. *Annals of Internal Medicine* **82,** 175.

Turner, D. J. and Wilson, J. (1969). The effect of diazepam on awareness during caesarean section under general anaesthesia. *British Medical Journal* **2,** 736.

Van der Kleijn, E., Van Rossum, J. M., Muskens, E. T. J. M. and Rijntijes, N. V. M. (1971). Pharmacokinetics of diazepam in dogs, mice and humans. *Acta pharmacologica et toxicologica* **29,** Suppl. 3, 109—27.

Wesseling, H. (1973). Comparative study of the efficacy of diazepam, pentobarbital and fentanyl-droperidol (Thalamonal) against toxicity induced by local anesthetics in mice. In: *The Benzodiazepines*, pp. 655—65. Ed. by S. Garattini, E. Mussini and L. O. Randall. Raven Press, New York.

Wilson, J. and Turner, D. J. (1969). Awareness during caesarean section under general anaesthesia. *British Medical Journal* **1,** 280.

Yeh, S. Y., Paul, R. H., Cordero, L. and Hon, E. H. (1974). A study of diazepam during labour. *Obstetrics and Gynecology* **43,** 363—73.

Zsigmond, E. K. and Shiveley, J. C. (1966). Spirometric and blood gas studies on the respiratory effects of hydroxyzine hydrochloride in the human volunteer. *Journal of New Drugs* **6,** 128.

8

Hypersensitivity reactions

R. S. J. Clarke

Thiopentone had been in clinical use from 1934 but it was not until 1952 that the first conclusive case of an allergic or hypersensitivity reaction occurred (Evans and Gould, 1952). Before this time and for many years after, writers had stated that such a condition did not exist, but since then the number of reports in the literature has increased steadily. At first these reports applied only to thiopentone but, as other intravenous anaesthetics came on the market, reactions to them were also described, and soon these overshadowed those due to the older drug. The numbers of published reports are shown in Fig. 8.1, and the recent progressive increase is striking. As there are presumably many unpublished reports and we have no way of knowing whether the increase in publications reflects a true increase in the

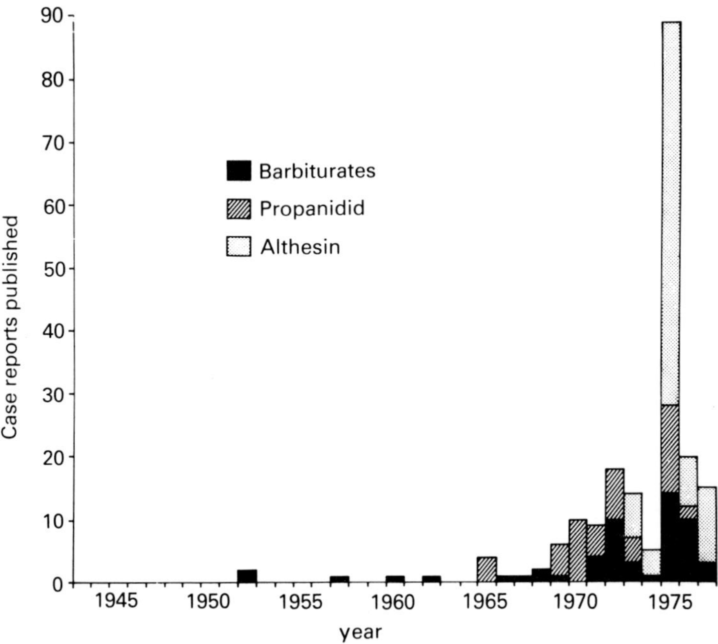

Fig. 8.1 Number of published cases of hypersensitivity reactions to the principal intravenous anaesthetics, 1943—1977.

incidence or only a higher proportion of them being reported. The latter seems more likely although it can be argued that as the general population takes more and more drugs annually, they are more likely to become cross-sensitized to a variety of pharmacological groups (Fisher, 1977a). Another possibility is that the chance of an individual having a repeat dose of a particular drug rises and, hence, the likelihood of an acquired hypersensitivity reaction. In support of this is the fact that Harrfeldt (1973) in West Germany had no reactions with propanidid in the first 35 000 administrations but 4 in the next 45 000.

Clinical manifestations

Contact dermatitis

This form of drug sensitivity should be considered before the generalized systemic reactions, if only to highlight the differences. It is perhaps surprising that there have been no reports of this problem in anaesthetists using any drug other than propanidid and indeed only two attributable to this agent (Sneddon and Glew, 1973; Dundee *et al.*, 1974).

Both anaesthetists developed intense itching and swelling of the eyelids and face so that vision became difficult. There was a similar but less marked effect on the hands and arms and the effect recurred with repeated exposures. In both cases there was some difficulty in defining the causative agent because it was not even necessary for the anaesthetist to give the anaesthetic — simply being in the same room was sufficient to cause the response. Spontaneous recovery was the usual course but in one case hydrocortisone 1 per cent cream and in the other chlorpheniramine maleate appeared to accelerate recovery. The face was most severely affected, presumably because of the fine droplets of propanidid dispersed either when filling a syringe and clearing it of bubbles or when the patient coughed during intubation. Patch tests in both cases showed sensitivity to propanidid but not to the solvent, cremophor, nor to Althesin which has the same solvent. Propanidid is a derivative of eugenol, which is related to oil of cloves, and contact dermatitis to this substance has been described in dental surgeons. Happily, this problem has not arisen with other intravenous anaesthetics and, since propanidid passed out of common use, desensitization has not been necessary.

Generalized reactions

The generalized reactions of which reports have been published are summarized in Tables 8.1 to 8.4. As many reports as could be traced have been included but the list may still not be complete. The reaction has been attributed to the intravenous induction agent administered; however, many patients also received a myoneural blocking drug. In the absence of skin testing this attribution may be wrong (Fisher, 1976a, b) but where sensitivity tests suggested a response to a relaxant the case has been omitted. Even if all tests were negative, cases have still been included if the clinical picture

Table 8.1 Generalized reactions to thiopentone, reported 1952—1977, with their clinical features and past history where known

Reference	No.	Clinical features				History			Deaths
		Skin	CVS	Broncho-spasm	GI	Atopy	Allergy	Same anaesthetic	
Evans and Gould (1952)	2	2	—	—	1	—	—	2	—
Hayward and Kiester (1957)	1	1	—	1	—	—	1	—	—
Kivalo, Wist and Mustakallio (1960)	1	1	1	1	1	—	1	—	—
Strunk (1962)	1	1	1	—	—	—	—	1	—
Currie *et al*. (1966)	1	1	1	1	—	—	1	1	—
Carrie and Buchanan (1967)	1	1	1	—	—	—	1	1	—
Anderton and Hopton (1968)	1	1	1	—	—	—	1	1	—
Cole (1968)	1	1	1	—	1	—	1	—	—
Clark and Cockburn (1971)	1	1	1	1	1	—	—	1	—
Davis (1971)	1	1	1	1	—	—	1	—	—
Fox, Wilkinson and Rabow (1971)	1	1	1	—	—	—	1	1	—
Holmes, Ross and Williams (1971)	1	1	1	1	—	—	1	—	1
Barjenbruch and Jones (1972)	1	1	1	—	—	—	1	1	—
Unsworth (1972)	2	2	2	1	—	—	2	2	—
Kelly and Boman (1973)	1	1	1	1	—	—	—	1	—
Wedley (1973)	1	—	—	1	—	—	—	—	—
Dundee *et al*. (1974)	1	1	1	1	—	1	1	1	—
Brown (1975)	1	—	1	—	—	—	—	1	—
Clarke *et al*. (1975)	12	8	8	10	—	5	3	5	4
Callens and Doutriaux (1976)	1	1	1	—	—	—	—	—	—
Guilmet and Joue (1976)	1	1	1	—	—	—	1	1	—
Laxenaire *et al*. (1976)	5	4	2	1	1	3	1	—	—
Saint-Maurice *et al*. (1976)	2	2	2	—	—	—	2	1	—
Stieglitz, Jacquot and Riondel (1976)	1	—	1	1	—	—	—	—	1
Evans and Keogh (1977)	3	2	3	2	—	—	2	—	—
Total	45	36	34	24	5	9	22	21	6

Table 8.2 Generalized reactions to barbiturates other than thiopentone, reported 1969—1977, with their clinical features and past history where known

Reference	No.	Clinical features				History			Deaths
		Skin	CVS	Broncho-spasm	GI	Atopy	Allergy	Same anaesthetic	
Methohexitone									
Shafto (1969)	1	—	1	—	—	—	—	—	—
Driggs and O'Day (1972)	6	6	6	5	3	3	1	—	—
Reichert and Basset (1972)	1	1	—	—	1	—	—	—	—
Wyatt and Watkins (1975)	1	—	—	—	—	—	—	—	—
Thiamylal									
Thompson, Eason and Flacke (1973)	1	1	1	1	—	—	—	—	—
Total	10	8	8	6	4	3	1	—	—

Table 8.3 Generalized reactions to propanidid, reported 1965—1977, with their clinical features and past history where known

Reference	No.	Clinical features				History			Deaths
		Skin	CVS	Broncho-spasm	GI	Atopy	Allergy	Same anaesthetic	
Beck (1965)	2	2	1	—	—	—	—	1	—
Radnay (1965)	1	1	1	—	—	—	—	—	—
Zindler (1965)	1	1	1	—	—	—	—	1	—
Gjessing (1969)	1	—	1	—	—	—	—	—	—
Kay (1969)	2	2	2	1	—	—	—	1	—
Manz and Frank (1969)	2	2	2	—	—	—	—	2	—
Bradburn (1970)	1	1	1	—	—	—	—	1	—
Dannemann and Lubke (1970)	2	2	2	—	—	—	—	2	—
Desai (in Johns, 1970)	1	1	1	—	1	—	—	1	—
Evans (1971)	1	1	1	—	—	—	—	—	—
Johns (1970)	1	1	1	—	—	—	—	1	—
Kruger (1970)	2	1	2	—	—	—	—	2	—
Larard (1970)	1	1	1	—	—	—	—	—	1
Miloschewsky and Cervenkova (1970)	1	1	1	—	—	—	—	—	—
Spreadbury and Marrett (1971)	1	1	1	—	—	—	—	—	—
Stovner and Endresen (1971)	3	3	3	—	—	—	—	3	1
Thornton (1971)	1	1	1	—	1	—	1	1	—
Gotla (1972)	1	1		—	1	—	—	—	—
Jarvis (1972)	1	1	1	—		—	1	1	—
Lorenz *et al.* (1972)	4	4	3	2	1	—	—	3	—
Rosenkranz (1972)	1	1	1	—	—	—	—	—	—
Turner, Keep and Batholomaeus (1972)	1	—	1	—	—	—	—	—	—
Harrfeldt (1973)	4	4	4	—	—	—	—	—	—
Clarke *et al.* (1975)	4	4	4	—	1	—	—	3	—
Doenicke (1975)	10	10	10	5	—	—	4	8	—
Laxenaire *et al.* (1976)	2	2	2	1	—	—	—	—	—
Total	52	49	49	9	5	0	6	31	2

Table 8.4 Generalized reactions to Althesin, reported 1973—1977, with their clinical features and past history where known*

Reference	No.	Clinical features				History			Deaths
		Skin	CVS	Broncho-spasm	GI	Atopy	Allergy	Same anaesthetic	
Avery and Evans (1973)	1	1	—	1	—	—	—	—	—
Crowther (1973)	1	—	—	1	—	—	—	1	—
Healy (1973)	1	—	—	1	—	—	—	1	—
Hester (1973)	1	1	1	1	—	—	—	—	—
Horton (1973)	1	1	1	—	—	—	—	1	—
Mehta (1973)	1	1	1	—	—	—	1	—	—
Notcutt (1973)	1	1	1	—	—	—	—	—	—
Dundee *et al*. (1974)	1	1	1	—	—	1	1	1	—
Kessell and Assem (1974)	1	1	1	—	—	1	—	—	—
Tweedie and Ordish (1974)	2	2	2	2	—	—	—	—	—
Clarke *et al*. (1975)	65	42	43	32	—	6	13	30	—
Bussien, Rybaric and Thurler (1975)	1	—	—	1	—	—	1	—	—
Fisher (1975)	2	2	2	—	2	—	—	2	—
Watt (1975)	4	2	4	3	—	—	—	3	—
Boytell (1976)	1	1	1	—	—	—	—	1	—
Fisher (1976a)	2	2	2	—	2	—	—	2	—
Laxenaire *et al*. (1976)	1	—	1	1	—	1	—	—	—
Monteil *et al*. (1976)	2	2	2	—	—	—	—	—	—
Rawicz, Rondio and Cwizewicz-Adamska (1976)	1	1	1	—	—	—	1	—	—
Steel (1976)	1	1	1	1	—	—	—	1	—
Callens and Doutriaux (1976)	1	1	1	1	—	—	—	—	—
Evans and Keogh (1977)	10	8	9	4	1	—	1	3	—
Total	91	62	67	43	5	7	16	42	—

*The findings in the first 10 reports are also included in the survey by Clarke *et al*. (1975)

Table 8.5 Unpublished reports of reactions to thiopentone, methohexitone, propanidid and Althesin which have reached the Department of Anaesthetics, The Queen's University of Belfast or Glaxo Laboratories, May 1975—December 1977 (i.e. after the period covered by the report by Clarke *et al.*, 1975)

Drug	No.	Clinical features				History			Deaths
		Skin	CVS	Broncho-spasm	GI	Atopy	Allergy	Same anaesthetic	
Thiopentone	22	15	19	15	2	5	7	8	1
Methohexitone	2	1	2	1	0	0	0	0	0
Propanidid	1	1	1	1	0	0	0	1	1
Althesin	111	87	91	51	3	9	15	60	3

followed the typical pattern. There was a particular difficulty with the reports of the meeting at Nancy, France, in 1975 because the same cases appeared in several papers (e.g. Laxenaire *et al.*, 1976; Vignon, Gay and Laxenaire, 1976), but as far as possible repetition has been avoided. Many patients were not questioned about past history of atopy, allergy or anaesthesia so the figures given are underestimates of these relationships.

Table 8.5 summarizes a further group of unpublished reports which have reached Glaxo Laboratories or the author. These cover the period May 1974 to December 1977 and cannot yet be regarded as complete. They do, however, indicate that the same type of reaction is continuing to occur and that those published separately by the anaesthetist concerned form only a small proportion of reactions actually occurring.

Cutaneous signs

These are discussed without distinguishing between causative drugs, since scrutiny of several hundred reports reveals no clear pattern differentiating the response to the various intravenous anaesthetics. There are two types of cutaneous reaction to intravenous drugs: one localized to the area of injection and the other, generalized. The localized reaction, along and around the vein of injection, is rare, unlike the reaction to pethidine which often produces a perivenous flare and wealing. Alleged cases must be scrutinized carefully because irritation due to perivenous injection of thiopentone is not uncommon but is usually distinguished by localized pain. This is a possible explanation of the case of Sargent (1971). A generalized cutaneous flush is much more common. This type of reaction occurs with tubocurarine in as many as 50 per cent of patients (McDowell and Clarke, 1969) and in 10—20 per cent with Althesin. It was described as early as 1943 by Davison but, because of the frequency of its occurrence, it is difficult to regard it as pathological. The bullous eruptions developing over several days described by Hunter (1943) and T. Fisher (1968), while allergic in origin, are also a different phenomenon. Cases of this type have not been included in Tables 8.1 to 8.4. Other cutaneous signs such as pilo-erection and blotchy urticaria do suggest a generalized hypersensitivity reaction.

Erythema, together with generalized oedema particularly of the eyelids, is a classical and common manifestation of hypersensitivity (Larard, 1970; Spreadbury and Marrett, 1971). Some of these patients also developed massive weals (Davis, 1971). When the element of oedema is present, it can be calculated that a 1 mm layer of subcutaneous fluid throughout the body represents a circulatory loss of about 1.5 litres. In fact this is very close to the fluid loss calculated from the haemoconcentration by Fisher (1977b). Visible oedema requires a much thicker fluid deposit and, though it is often unevenly spread, it is not hard to see how hypotension and circulatory failure can result. The most serious form is oedema of the glottis; but only in a few instances has this been definitely reported. However, many of the reports of coughing, difficulty in breathing and laryngospasm (Clarke *et al.*, 1975) may have been due to incipient laryngeal oedema.

In general, the skin colour has been described as bright red or, if there was also peripheral circulatory failure, as cyanosed. These reactions, with or without cardiovascular signs, have been classified as 'histaminoid' because the effects closely resemble those of histamine release. However, in a small proportion of patients there was marked cutaneous pallor sometimes preceded by flushing or cyanosis but accompanied by oedema and/or severe hypotension. These have been classified as 'cardiovascular collapse' (Clarke *et al.*, 1975) and, although they are hard to include in the same group as histaminoid they should probably be regarded as another manifestation of hypersensitivity. They are therefore included in the 'histaminoid' group in the Tables. Sometimes clear reactions have occurred 12—80 minutes after administration of the drug (Clarke *et al.*, 1975; Callens and Doutriaux, 1976; Laxenaire *et al.*, 1976) and these have also been included with the main group.

Cardiovascular changes

Hypotension accompanies the widespread capillary vasodilation in the majority of hypersensitivity reactions and is accentuated by the transudation of fluid into the tissue spaces. This is accompanied by tachycardia which is probably a reflex response to the hypotension. The severe hypotension, even if it is described clinically as a 'cardiac arrest', often returns to normal spontaneously as compensatory mechanisms come into play. There is no reason to postulate any direct cardiac involvement. In patients treated actively, administration of intravenous fluids is probably the most useful measure to restore the blood pressure to normal. Ventricular fibrillation is rare and cardiostimulatory drugs appear to have only a secondary place in the management of the collapse.

Bronchospasm

This is the most frequent feature of hypersensitivity reactions, whether on its own or as an accompaniment to cardiovascular changes. In clinical practice the word is often used as a first diagnosis for any unexplained airway obstruction, including a blocked endotracheal tube or herniated cuff. Even if confirmed, however, it is still difficult for the anaesthetist to be certain whether this is due to irritation of the larynx by saliva or gastric juice, or by a laryngoscope or endotracheal tube if these have been introduced. Certainly these factors must be excluded before a diagnosis of hypersensitivity is accepted. Other symptoms and signs of a more clearly defined nature help to confirm the diagnosis. Severe bronchospasm, particularly if accompanied by hypotension, leads rapidly to cerebral hypoxia and this combination has been responsible for most of the deaths which have occurred. Under the same heading may be included copious production of mucus from the bronchial tree, which often accompanies bronchospasm, but again other causative factors must be excluded.

Other effects

Abdominal pain and vomiting are more rare manifestations but are certainly associated with some reactions (Cole, 1968; Clarke *et al.*, 1975). Delay in recovery in consciousness has been noted (Currie *et al.*, 1966; Clark and Cockburn, 1971; Unsworth, 1972) but only with thiopentone. On the other hand, reactions have occurred during recovery from anaesthesia with propanidid. It does not therefore seem likely that the delay is a part of the reaction; more probably, it is a consequence of a poor local circulation.

Natural course

The exact order of events is variable but usually the first sign to attract attention is a flush or cough. The skin may become cyanosed and breathing difficult because of the bronchospasm or laryngospasm. The pulse, when felt, is rapid and weak, soon becoming impalpable. Should such a reaction occur in the sitting position (in a dentist's chair) or be left untreated, it may lead to ventricular fibrillation although the majority of patients probably have no more than severe hypotension and recover with minimal treatment (see below).

Differential diagnosis

The most important differential diagnosis of hypersensitivity is overdosage. This may be actual or relative to the health of the patient. For many years now the common induction dose of thiopentone has been 4—5 mg·kg^{-1} and, provided it is reduced in conditions such as hypovolaemic shock, old age and indeed severe illness of any kind, there is little danger of overdosage. The same is not true of propanidid and Althesin. Propanidid can be shown to be virtually equipotent with thiopentone (Clarke *et al.*, 1968) but, because of its short duration of action, doses of 6—8 mg·kg^{-1} are often given. Although both drugs are myocardial depressants and cause peripheral vasodilatation, the side effects of propanidid become more marked as the dose rises. This is because the dose/toxicity curve of propanidid is steeper than that of thiopentone (Clarke and Dundee, 1970). In addition, Soga and his colleagues (1973) compared propanidid with a barbiturate and found it to be more depressant to the myocardium. Soon after the appearance of the first reports of collapse following propanidid, the suggestion was made of possible overdosage (Clarke and Dundee, 1969), and Grimmeisen (1971) and Zindler (1975) have supported this view. This is not the whole explanation, and Doenicke has (1975) confirmed this from an analysis of dose against frequency of incidence of reactions to propanidid. The most frequently administered adult dose was 500 mg and no severe reactions occurred with this dose. Neither the occurrence rate nor the severity of reaction appears to be dose-dependent.

Early studies with Althesin indicated that 50 μl·kg^{-1} was approximately equipotent with thiopentone 4 mg·kg^{-1} (Carson, Dundee and Clarke, 1975). It had a high therapeutic index in animals (Child *et al.*, 1971) and man (Clarke, Dundee and Carson, 1972), causing little hypotension or myocardial depression in doses up to 150 μl·kg^{-1}. However, the small dose volume of Althesin as marketed compared with 2.5 per cent thiopentone does encourage overdosage and too rapid administration. The dose required to induce anaesthesia is more variable with Althesin than with the barbiturates (Carson, Dundee and Clarke, 1975), and Mathieu and Grilliat (1976) believe that dose and rate of injection are factors in anaphylactoid reactions to Althesin. Certainly several authors have reported a reduced incidence and less severe hypotension with slow administration (Samuel and Dundee, 1973; Fantera and Maurina, 1976). Sutton (1976) also made suggestions of a similar nature.

Overdosage is a likely cause of profound hypotension during induction but it is very unlikely to cause erythema, oedema, weals or bronchospasm. It is therefore in the patients presenting with marked pallor and cardiovascular collapse that overdose should be seriously considered.

Other syndromes can cause collapse and acute intermittent porphyria (with barbiturates), pulmonary embolism and myocardial infarction, and carcinoid tumour must be remembered (Clark and Cockburn, 1971). Gastric aspiration is probably the commonest cause of bronchospasm during induction of anaesthesia and can only be confirmed by testing the acidity of fluid aspirated from a tracheal tube with litmus paper.

Mechanism

Role of histamine

The clinical events described closely resemble the known effects of histamine in man, which may perhaps be summarized here. There is a profound dilatation of the capillaries in all vascular beds but particularly in the skin of the upper half of the body (Dale and Laidlaw, 1919). There is also an increase in capillary permeability although Douglas (1975) stressed that these changes occur not only in the capillaries but in the whole range of vessels from terminal arteriole to small venule. The vessels become permeable to plasma proteins, as shown by studies with attached dyes such as Evans blue, and this accentuates the fluid loss. Dilatation of the cerebral vessels leads to severe headache which has been attributed to stretching of the sensory endings around the cranial arteries. Histamine has little direct action on the heart but failure of the venous return lowers the cardiac output. Tachycardia is probably due to sympathetic stimulation and release of adrenaline from the adrenal medulla.

Contraction, or even spasm, of the smooth muscle of the intestine is another direct action of histamine. Bronchoconstriction following histamine administration is not normally severe in man but patients suffering from asthma are more seriously affected. Finally, a fall in basophil count and increased production of gastric acid can be demonstrated.

Plasma histamine levels

The resemblance between an adverse reaction to an intravenous anaesthetic and the actions of histamine described above is very close but it is only in the last ten years that measurements of plasma histamine during an anaphylactoid episode have been made. There appear to be two distinct types of histamine release caused by anaesthetic and other drugs. The first is the release of very small amounts (1–4 $\mu g \cdot l^{-1}$). This occurs in the great majority of patients following the administration of thiopentone, propanidid and Althesin but not etomidate or Cremophor EL (Lorenz *et al.*, 1972; Doenicke *et al.*, 1973). This histamine release is increased by high

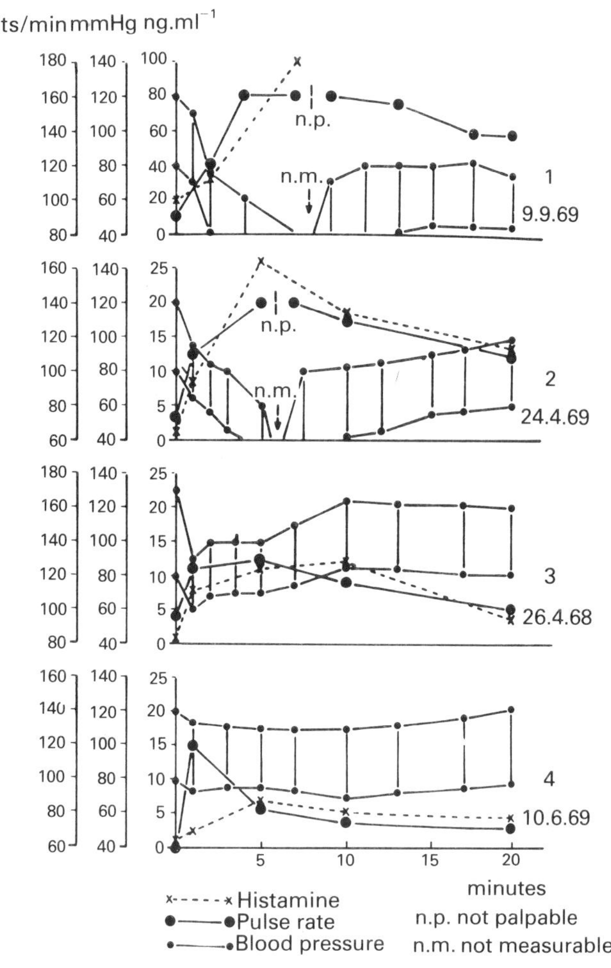

Fig. 8.2 Heart rate, blood pressure and plasma histamine concentration in 4 patients with anaphylactoid reactions to propanidid. (From Lorenz *et al.*, 1972.)

dosage and rapid injection, and by hypoxia, hypercarbia and acidosis (co-liberators) (Mongar and Schild, 1962). It may contribute to the hypotension which is a feature of intravenous induction of anaesthesia but on the whole it seems to be unrelated to the phenomenon of hypersensitivity. However, there must be a range of histamine liberation in patients; a few have a massive direct histamine release which is clinically indistinguishable from the hypersensitivity reaction but the patients do not have a positive response to sensitivity tests. The existence of this group is particularly stressed by the French and German workers but, because of the unreliability of sensitivity tests (see below), it is convenient to include them in figures for true reactions. Lorenz and his colleagues (1972) also studied four patients during anaphylactoid reactions to propanidid and found a close correlation between plasma histamine level and clinical manifestations. The two patients with the severe reactions (systolic BP <40 mmHg; HR >140; widespread erythema; bronchospasm) had plasma histamine levels of 26—100 $\mu g \cdot l^{-1}$ (Fig. 8.2). The two patients with trivial reactions of similar type had levels of 6—12 $\mu g \cdot l^{-1}$. There have been no similar studies during anaphylactoid reactions to other anaesthetics but it seems likely that, with all of them, histamine is the final mediator.

Immune mechanisms

Information is now accumulating on the events preceding the histamine liberation phase. Blood samples have been obtained from many patients having alleged anaphylactoid reactions and the immunoglobulins and complement analysed (Watkins *et al.*, 1976b). It is apparent from two-dimensional immunoelectrophoresis that, following an adverse reaction, complement factors C3 and C4 are consumed. C3 is converted first to C3b and then to C3c while C3a is also generated (Fig. 8.3). This may be expressed as percentage conversion of C3 which is maximal in the early hours after a reaction but later returns towards normal. The time course appears to differ after reactions to Althesin and the barbiturates, recovery taking about 24 hours after the former and 72 hours following thiopentone or methohexitone reactions. It is the very active polypeptide C3a (anaphylatoxin) which is probably responsible for the histamine liberation.

One of the advances to emerge from these studies is that we now have a biochemical test which will distinguish, in retrospect, a true hypersensitivity reaction from an overdose or other anaesthetic mishap. It does involve obtaining early serial samples at (say) 2, 6, 12 and 24 hours and 5 days, separating off the plasma and storing it, preferably at —20°C, until analysed.

Another approach to the problem has been the serial analysis of the leucocytes and, in particular, the lymphocytes after induction of anaesthesia. Watkins and his colleagues (1976a) have shown that about 50 per cent of patients have a significant change in white cell types and numbers. The pattern is fairly consistent, with a sharp rise of about 25 per cent over the first 10 minutes following the administration of the drug and a return to normal within a further 10 minutes. A similar percentage of patients

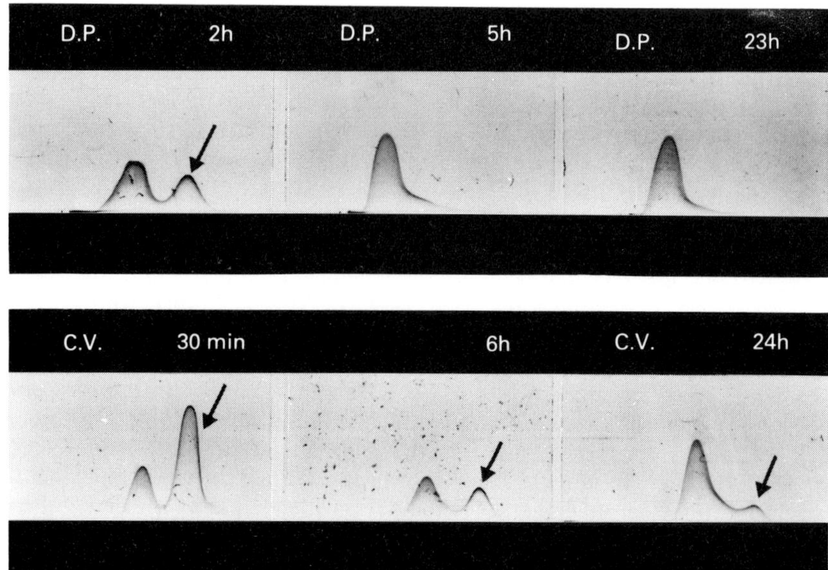

Fig. 8.3 Two-dimensional immunoelectrophoresis patterns of C3 component in plasma samples taken from patients DP and CV, respectively. Times after Althesin induction are indicated. The first dimension electrophoresis was carried out towards the right of the illustration; the C3 conversion product (C3c, indicated by arrows) possesses greater electrophoretic mobility than *native* C3. The difference in degree of conversion exhibited by these patients reflects the difference in clinical severity of the adverse response: the surgical procedure had to be abandoned in the case of CV. (From Watkins, Udnoon and Taussig, 1978.)

receiving the drug on a subsequent occasion had a significant drop in the leucocyte count over the same period. These observations were made following Althesin, propanidid and methohexitone. Immunoelectrophoresis studies carried out at the same time showed that there was a small amount (10 per cent) of complement conversion on the first induction but that the degree of conversion was much greater and more prolonged on the second induction. In addition, it was demonstrated in one volunteer who showed this reaction that sodium cromoglycate reversed the fall in lymphocyte count.

Cremophor EL

Propanidid and the components of Althesin (alphaxalone and alphadolone acetate) are sparingly soluble in water. The organic solvent Cremophor EL has therefore been used to facilitate their dispensing in solutions of reasonable volume. In fact, this is not a pure substance but has hydrophylic and hydrophobic components; the molecular weight of the latter can only be given as approximately 3170 at 37°C (Scholtan and Lie, 1966). The LD_{50} is 6500 mg·kg^{-1} in the mouse and 640 mg·kg^{-1} in the dog, its toxicity in the latter animal being related to histamine liberation. Many studies have shown that it does not cause cardiovascular depression (Savege, Foley and Simpson, 1973) or histamine liberation in man (Lorenz *et al.*, 1972; Doenicke *et al.*, 1973). It is quickly eliminated, principally by the kidneys (Duhm *et al.*, 1965). The formulation of Cremophor EL was changed about 1969 but records of heart rate changes and miscellaneous side effects showed no difference between the two preparations of propanidid (Doenicke, 1975). There is also no evidence of local or generalised sensitivity to Cremophor EL on its own. Anaesthetists with a skin sensitivity to propanidid have been able to use Althesin without trouble (Sneddon and Glew, 1973; Dundee *et al.*, 1974). It does not cause leucocyte degranulation in patients in whom propanidid or Althesin produce this effect (Watkins *et al.*, 1976a).

Evidence against Cremophor EL is still indefinite. For instance, Notcutt (1973) described a reaction to Althesin two weeks after exposure to propanidid. Kessell and Assem (1974) described a case of anaphylaxis to Althesin in a patient who was sensitive to Althesin, propanidid and Cremophor on skin testing. At least 5 patients out of 70 having reactions following Althesin (Tweedie and Ordish, 1974; Clarke *et al.*, 1975) had been previously exposed to propanidid. It has been suggested by Watkins and his colleagues (1976a) that the surfactant properties of Cremophor EL may enhance the immunogenicity of both propanidid and Althesin; until experiments prove or disprove this theory, it appears to be the most likely interpretation of the observations.

Diazepam in the usual formulation, dissolved in propylene glycol, benzoic acid and sodium benzoate, causes a high incidence of pain on intravenous injection, and venous thrombosis. Attempts have therefore been made to use Cremophor EL as a solvent (Stesolid). Unfortunately, the change to this preparation in Scandinavia, though reducing the amount of pain on injection, has led to a high incidence of anaphylactoid reactions. Even in the absence of a detailed study to investigate the cause of the reactions, the newer preparation has been almost abandoned.

Summary of the mechanism

It appears that in anaphylactoid reactions to intravenous induction agents there are three distinct mechanisms. First, there is the direct pharmacological effect of the drug, causing in the majority of individuals some release of histamine from basophils. This can occur on the first or subsequent exposures to a drug and, while the quantity is usually small, it will be highly dependent on dose and rate of injection. Secondly, there is chemical activation of the complement C3 to undergo conversion with a simultaneous rise in leucocyte count. This can occur by means of the so-called 'alternate pathway' and does not involve IgE or immune recognition, i.e. previous exposure to the drug. This is clearly a very common phenomenon with many drugs but only rarely does it lead to a major liberation of histamine into the blood stream with a catastrophic reaction. The third possibility is that a patient who has been previously exposed to a drug has built up IgE antibodies to it. These antibodies become bound to mast cells or to basophils. Subsequent challenge with the specific antigen results in immune recognition by the IgE receptors resulting in immediate histamine release from the cells which again may be trivial or may provoke a typical anaphylactic attack. There may then be secondary complement C3 conversion, so that its estimation does not distinguish between these two mechanisms. In this type of phenomenon there is typically a fall in leucocyte count.

Incidence of reactions and deaths with different drugs

It has been stressed that the phenomena described are not specific for a particular drug and there is no clinical pattern distinguishing between the different agents concerned. Figures for any hypersensitivity reaction (other than a simple skin rash) are around 1 in 5000 to 1 in 8000 (Fisher, 1975; Laxenaire *et al.*, 1976; Evans and Keogh, 1977). However, there have been considerable differences in the incidence reported between different drugs and between different series.

Barbiturates

There are few incidence figures for thiopentone although Evans and Keogh (1977) in their Cardiff series give a figure of 1 in 29 000 and Shaw (1974) reports 1 in 36 000 in New Zealand. Both are admitted to be underestimates. There are, all together, reports of 45 authentic reactions including 6 deaths (Table 8.1). In addition, there has been one reported reaction to thiamylal (Thompson, Eason and Flacke, 1973). The only actual estimate of reactions to methohexitone is that of Driggs and O'Day (1972). They described 6 cases from one dental clinic in California, giving an incidence of about 1 in 7000 in their practice (with no deaths). Although this is obviously an over-estimate, the total of 9 reported cases shows that reactions following this agent are not as rare as is often supposed. We have records of 22 000 administrations in the Musgrave Park Hospital, Belfast, with no reactions. A much reported case of an adverse reaction to methohexitone (Shafto, 1969) occurred in a child who had previously fainted while awaiting the dental anaesthetic.

Propanidid

It was the incidence of reactions following propanidid which first alarmed anaesthetists, and earlier figures for this drug range from Danneman and Lubke's (1970) 4 in 3000 to Kay's (1972) 3 in 5000. Comparing these figures with Table 8.3 it is clear that, although there have been few published case reports of adverse reactions to this drug, there have been very many episodes indicated only by numbers (Werner and Wolff, 1970). The analysis by Doenicke (1975) reports about 1 reaction in 170 administrations, and

Harrfeldt (1973) reports fewer than 1 in 10 000. The rate is probably too high for acceptability but it must still be considered that the known deaths do not indicate that it is a very dangerous drug.

Althesin

The total of published reactions following the use of this drug has now reached 91 and many more reports are known to the author, but this large number of reports is mainly due to the attitude of the manufacturers in collecting the reports and encouraging their detailed study. In Northern Ireland the author has records of 4000 consecutive Althesin anaesthetics from 1970 to 1973 with no reactions, though there have been 17 since the latter date because the drug was more freely used. The figures for incidence based on reported reactions and the known sales of the drug are about 1 in 11 000 inductions (Clarke *et al.*, 1975). If cases in which a muscle relaxant was used are not included, the incidence becomes 1 in 19 000 inductions. Compared with these relatively low figures, derived from retrospective follow-up with voluntary reporting, there are also three reports of studies in circumscribed hospital groups. Watt (1975) in England reported 1 in 900; Fisher (1976a) from Wellington, New Zealand, an incidence of 1 in 900; and Evans and Keogh (1977) reported 1 in 1900 in Cardiff, Wales. The three groups come from differing areas using different batches of the drug so it is difficult to blame these factors for the higher incidence. On the other hand, our own continuing (unpublished) survey still indicates an overall reaction rate of about 1 in 10 000. Fisher (1976a) has drawn attention to this clash of evidence for which he has no satisfactory explanation.

Mortality attributable to Althesin reactions in the UK is still very low. Four deaths are known to have occurred, of which 1 was probably due to the poor health of the patient (Avery and Evans, 1973) and 1 (unpublished) was probably not directly caused by Althesin. In the other 2, intractable bronchospasm was certainly the main clinical feature of the reaction but suxamethonium was also used in one of these patients.

Muscle relaxants

These have been involved in reports of anaesthetic morbidity almost since their introduction. Drugs involved include gallamine (Lopert, 1955; Walmsley, 1959; Hainsworth and Bingham, 1970), suxamethonium (Kepes and Haimovici, 1959; Jerums, Whittingham and Wilson, 1967; Katz and Mulligan, 1972), tubocurarine (Comroe and Dripps, 1946; Salem, Kim and El Etr, 1968; Westgate, Schultz and Van Bergen, 1961) and alcuronium (Chan and Yeung, 1972). Pancuronium liberates only minimal amounts of histamine (Buckett, 1968) but bronchospasm has still occurred (Clark, 1973; Heath, 1973). More recently, Fisher (1975, 1976b) has described positive intradermal tests to suxamethonium, gallamine and tubocurarine, and Vervloet and his colleagues (1977) have shown a high incidence of positive tests to some dilutions of the muscle relaxants in the patients studied. It cannot be assumed therefore that, where an induction agent was immediately followed by a relaxant, the former was alone responsible for any adverse reaction. Even when bronchospasm following tracheal intubation is discounted, it is clear from reports that the general features of bronchospasm, hypotension and oedema are very similar to those following the intravenous anaesthetics.

Reactions to other drugs used by the anaesthetist are also frequent. Penicillin anaphylactoid reactions have an incidence of between 1 and 4 in 10 000, with a death rate of 1 in 50 000 (Idsøe *et al.*, 1968), and reactions have been reported under anaesthesia (Katz, Battit and Wilkey, 1970; Cullen, 1971). Three reactions to cephalothin during anaesthesia have been described, 2 of which were fatal (Spruill, Minette and Sturner, 1974; Velazquez and Gold, 1975). However, the plasma expanders probably cause more dangerous anaphylactoid reactions than any other agents used in anaesthesia. The total figures obtained by Ring and Messmer (1977) indicate reaction rates per 10 000 administrations of 1.4 for plasma proteins, 3.2 for dextrans, 8.5 for hydroxyethyl starch and 11.5 for gelatins. When it is considered that many of the patients receiving these products are already hypovolaemic, it must be concluded that starch and gelatin solutions are unacceptably dangerous.

Predisposing factors

Age and sex

There is no evidence that these factors have any bearing on the occurrence of hypersensitivity reactions. About one-third of the patients in the series of Clarke and his colleagues (1975) were under 20 and one-third were over 50. There was a slight preponderance of females in the middle group and of males in the older group, as one would expect from the distribution of gynaecological and urological surgery.

Atopy (asthma, hay fever and eczema)

The broad survey of reactions as mentioned above (Clarke *et al.*, 1975) indicated that 14 per cent of reactors had an atopic history. This is close to that in the general population (Halpern *et al.*, 1973; Pepys, 1973) but, in the absence of a specific study, it was not possible to decide whether this was also true for the surgical population. A survey was therefore carried out by The Queen's University of Belfast, of a range of anaesthetists throughout the British Isles. They were asked to complete questionnaires on the atopic, allergic and anaesthetic histories of their patients and 10 000 returns were analysed (Dundee *et al.*, 1978). The overall incidence in the 10 000 patients was: asthma 3.5 per cent; hay fever 3.8 per cent; eczema 2.4 per cent; any one of these 8.5 per cent. The incidence of any atopic history in the published cases (not all of whom were questioned regarding history) was only 9 per cent (Table 8.6). This difference is not statistically significant — that is, there is no demonstrable association between atopic history and hypersensitivity reactions to intravenous anaesthetics in general. However,

Table 8.6 Percentage of those reacting to various intravenous anaesthetics and of the general surgical population with history of atopy, allergies and exposure to one of the three anaesthetic groups

	Number	History of				
		Atopy	Allergy	Previous exposure to		
				Barbiturates	Propanidid	Althesin
Reactors to barbiturates (Tables 8.1 and 8.2)	55	22	42	38	—	—
Reactors to propanidid (Table 8.3)	52	0	12	—	56	—
Reactors to Althesin (Table 8.4)	91	7	15	—	—	46
Total of reactors	198	9	22	—	—	—
General surgical population*	10 000	8.5	13.5	53.6	—	12.1

*Figures from Dundee *et al*. (1978) and Fee *et al*. (1978)

there is a significant difference between the reactors to barbiturates and the general population ($\chi^2 = 12.38$; $P<0.0005$). The fact that no atopic history is recorded for any of the propanidid reactors is probably due to lack of questioning rather than a genuine difference in those reacting to barbiturates.

Allergy

A relationship between allergic history and drug reactions in general has been shown by Hurwitz (1969). The review of adverse reactions by Clarke and his colleagues (1975) revealed an allergic history in 20 per cent of these, and the more general survey gives a figure of 22 per cent (Table 8.6). The overall survey of surgical patients gave an incidence of only 13.5 per cent (Fee *et al.*, 1978) and this figure is significantly different from that in the published descriptions of reactions ($\chi^2 = 11.11$; $P<0.01$). The relationship is even more striking for the barbiturate reactors, 42 per cent of whom gave a history of allergy. There is also a highly significant association between atopy and allergy, so the two factors can be analysed together. When this is done (not shown in the Tables), there is a highly significant difference since 29.3 per cent of reactors have a history of atopy and/or allergy against 19.0 per cent of the general surgical population ($\chi^2 = 13.26$; $P>0.005$).

Doenicke's (1975) retrospective study of 2209 propanidid anaesthetics revealed a general incidence of 8.2 per cent of surgical patients having a history of allergy, against 15.6 per cent of patients reacting to propanidid who had a history of previous allergic manifestations.

Previous anaesthetics

An anaphylactoid reaction to any substance is often assumed to be due to sensitization by previous exposure to the same drug. This association has been demonstrated by Currie (1970) and by Hurwitz (1969). The figures in Table 8.6 show that about 50 per cent of those in each group of reactors are known to have had the same anaesthetic previously. These are minimum estimates, for in some patients the previous drug exposure history is not recorded or known. Comparable control figures for the drug exposure of the surgical population are difficult to obtain because we can only determine the percentage of patients known to have previously had an anaesthetic. This was determined by the above-mentioned survey and was surprisingly high, at 66.7 per cent (Fee *et al.*, 1978). Figure 8.4 shows an analysis of the 10 000 patients in terms of the number of previous anaesthetic exposures. The distribution of anaesthetic histories in the whole surgical population can be estimated from the distribution in the 2780 patients in whom it was known. The figures indicated that 80.4 per cent of patients previously anaesthetized had received thiopentone and 18.1 per cent had received Althesin. Estimated figures for the total surgical population are therefore 53.6 per cent for thiopentone and 12.1 per cent for Althesin. (Unfortunately, propanidid was not included in the survey.) The figure of 80 per cent for thiopentone is similar to that obtained in a previous survey of UK hospitals by Dundee (1956) and by Evans and Keogh (1977). Since the majority of patients who have had an anaesthetic have probably had an intravenous anaesthetic, it is likely that the distribution of exposure in the surgical population as a whole is as shown in the Table.

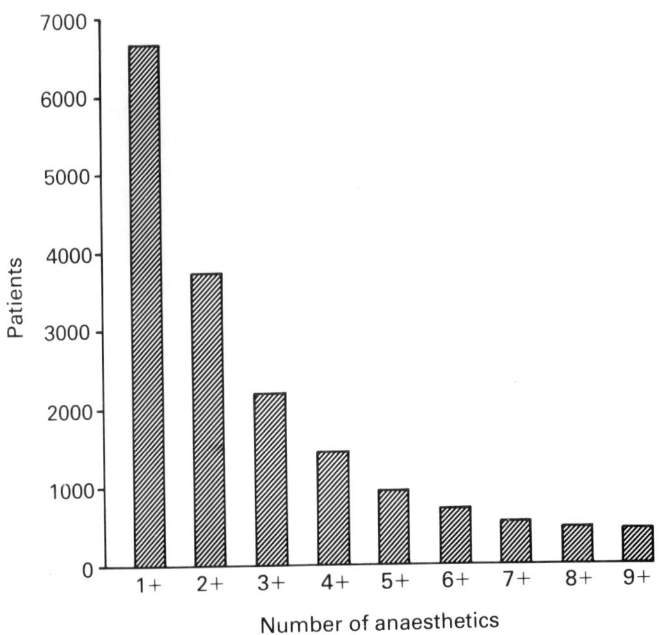

Fig. 8.4 Number of previous exposures to any general anaesthetic in a survey of 10 000 patients.

It therefore appears that a history of previous exposure is no more common in those having adverse reactions to thiopentone than in the general surgical population. Calculations regarding the other anaesthetics are more liable to error. The percentages of the general surgical population receiving the less common drugs are much lower than for thiopentone. Certainly they are much lower than the percentages of those having previous exposure in the reactor group. It does therefore seem likely that sensitization to propanidid and Althesin in particular is a true causative factor in inducing reactions to these drugs. This is also Doenicke's (1975) conclusion for propanidid since he found in a retrospective study that 22 per cent of the reactions occurred during first anaesthetics and 78 per cent during subsequent exposures.

It must also be stressed that about half of all adverse reactions occur in patients who have not previously been exposed to the same anaesthetic.

Investigative measures

When a patient has a severe reaction to an anaesthetic, there is clearly a need, not only to understand the reaction but also to identify the offending agent and warn the patient against it. Many anaesthetists have doubted the value of the usual type of intradermal test (Fox, Wilkinson and Rabow, 1971) because of the number of false positive and false negative reactions but many have used it for lack of a better test (Anderton and Hopton, 1968; Hainsworth and Bingham, 1970; Watt, 1975). Fisher (1976b) has stressed its value because of its simplicity and high yield of results provided that solutions are prepared freshly and dilutions of 1:1000 are used initially to avoid false positives. As far as can be safely demonstrated the test appears to detect the offending drug and those not incriminated can be given safely. There are, however, false positives, particularly with the myoneural blocking drugs, if not diluted (Vervloet *et al.*, 1977). Testing is unreliable at the extremes of age and anaphylactic reactions may be followed by a refractory period of 3–4 weeks so that an adequate interval should be allowed after a reaction before submitting a patient to skin testing. Sympathomimetic drugs, antihistamines and steroids may also inhibit a skin reaction.

The recommended test procedure is therefore to prepare fresh solutions of all drugs and solvents that are relevant, dilute them to 1 : 1000 and inject 0.1 ml intradermally on the anterior surface of the forearm after cleaning the skin with alcohol. A positive reaction is a flare with a weal of at least 1.5 cm appearing within 30 minutes and persisting for 30 minutes. If there is a reaction to more than one drug, both should be tested in a dilution of 1 : 10000. Fisher (1975) reported an instance where a dilution of 1 : 100 provoked a systemic reaction in a sensitive patient but he believes that with the more dilute solution the risk is small. Resuscitation facilities should, however, always be available. When testing with Althesin and cremophor a dilution of 1:100 gives more consistent results (Fisher, 1977b).

Other skin tests such as the patch and prick tests are probably valueless. The passive transfer of Prausnitz—Kuestner test is performed by injecting 0.1 ml of the patient's serum and serum from a normal control, intradermally into three or four sites in the forearm of two recipients (Currie, 1970). After 24 hours 0.1 ml of the drugs under test and controls are injected into the same area in similar dilutions to those used in the intradermal test. This test can be used to demonstrate the presence of an antibody to the drug (IgE) but it carries some risk of serum hepatitis and adds little to the results of simple intradermal testing.

In a leucocyte degranulation test (Kessell and Assem, 1974) the patients' basophils are challenged with the test drug and solvents and controls are examined for loss of histamine-containing granules. However, the test is time-consuming and requires a large amount of fresh blood.

Measurements of complement and immunoglobulins (IgA, IgF, IgM and IgE) can be made (Watkins *et al.*, 1976a, b) but, while they help to demonstrate a hypersensitivity reaction, they do not clearly identify the agent responsible.

Trial administration of the suspected drug has been used (Carrie and Buchanan, 1967; Lorenz *et al.*, 1972) but it is difficult to justify ethically. In addition, it is possible that patients could react adversely to a drug on one occasion and yet have an uneventful anaesthetic with the same drug subsequently. This has been suggested as the explanation of an episode of angioneurotic oedema which was demonstrated by leucocyte degranulation to be due to propanidid (or atropine), 17 weeks after the anaesthetic. However, 22 and 30 weeks after the episode the tests were negative. In a less striking case (Clarke *et al.*, 1975), a patient who had a marked flush following Althesin on one occasion had no reaction with a repeat demonstration.

The importance of all these factors, particularly in combination, is stressed by Moneret-Vautrin, Duc and Sigiel (1976).

Prevention

There does not appear to be any practicable way of preventing adverse reactions to intravenous anaesthetics but certainly the severity of miscellaneous anaesthetic incidents can be reduced by using moderate doses of all drugs and administering the dose slowly. The fact that such reactions are commoner in patients with an atopic or allergic history has little bearing on the choice of anaesthetic technique because almost all anaesthetic drugs can induce anaphylactoid reactions. However, there is evidence that propanidid and Althesin are followed by a higher incidence of reactions than thiopentone, so it is probably safer to restrict induction to thiopentone and methohexitone (but using ketamine and diazepam or a neurolept combination where they are indicated). Obviously, where a patient is known to have an allergy to a particular drug, it should be avoided, as should drugs of a similar molecular structure.

Premedication

Studies are now available from Germany showing that pretreatment with an antihistamine (clemastine) reduces both incidence and severity of adverse reactions (Lorenz *et al.*, 1972; Doenicke, 1975). Pretreatment with prednisolone or hydrocortisone also reduces the severity of reactions but this is clearly a measure which should not be employed routinely. Even the use of antihistamines has certain disadvantages, in particular causing an increase in the excitatory side effects following thiopentone or methohexitone (Dundee, 1965). Disodium cromoglycate can block the signs of immune recognition of Althesin *in vitro* (Watkins *et al.*, 1976a) but its clinical value has yet to be demonstrated.

Prevention of adverse reactions is not possible but a reduction of the hazards can be achieved by energetic treatment. Details of this will be discussed below but it is clearly essential that all intravenous inductions should be carried out in rooms equipped for positive pressure ventilation, intubation, massive intravenous infusion and administration of a range of drugs.

Treatment

The main components of the hypersensitivity reaction are vasodilatation and exudation of fluid into the tissue spaces. The reaction is very often self-limiting and spontaneous recovery occurs after some minutes. The most frequently employed and safest treatment is therefore to administer intravenous fluids, usually 500—2000 ml sodium lactate injection compound BP (Clarke *et al.*, 1975). Fisher (1977c) estimated the plasma loss as 1—2 litres and found that, as the replacement volume approached this figure, the degree of haemoconcentration was reduced. However, he has also shown that when electrolyte solutions were used the loss continued in spite of the infusion of large volumes, whereas when colloid solutions were infused the haemoconcentration was corrected. Fisher (1977c) administered a purified plasma protein solution but it is likely that dextran or gelatin solutions would be equally effective. He also suggested that with a severe reaction most of the intracellular histamine will have been released and there is little risk of a further reaction to the colloid solution. The urgent treatment of the hypotension is therefore to tilt the patient head down and to start an infusion, giving first colloid plasma expanders and later electrolyte solutions.

The management of the respiratory problems is by the administration of oxygen, tracheal intubation and, if necessary, positive pressure ventilation. Frequently the 'bronchospasm' is due to a mechanical airway obstruction and all the possible causes of obstruction must be checked. Obstruction in pharynx or larynx prior to intubation is easily treated and, even in the presence of laryngeal oedema, tracheal intubation is not too difficult.

The administration of antihistamines is only of value in the treatment of urticaria and angioneurotic oedema (chlorpheniramine 10 mg intravenously). However, as these signs develop late in many cases, Fisher (1975) recommends the routine use of antihistamines.

Drug treatment of bronchospasm should begin with a slow intravenous injection of aminophylline 250 mg. Adrenaline 1 : 1000 solution 0.3 ml may be given by intramuscular injection as treatment for both the bronchospasm and cardiovascular collapse. However, there is a risk that it will precipitate ventricular fibrillation if the heart is already hypoxic. The administration of peripherally acting vasoconstrictors such as metaraminol and methoxamine in divided doses should be considered while the blood pressure is low and before the plasma volume has been fully expanded. Hydrocortisone 100—500 mg or a related steroid is probably beneficial to counteract both bronchospasm and hypotension (Lorenz *et al.*, 1972). It is, however, not of immediate benefit in the acute emergency.

Continued observation and supportive treatment will probably be necessary and the patient should be admitted to an intensive care unit. Infusions of adrenaline or isoprenaline may be needed to maintain an adequate circulation; tracheal intubation will ensure a good airway and ventilation with a high oxygen concentration may be required to combat the pulmonary oedema.

References

Anderton, J. M. and Hopton, D. S. (1968). Thiopentone anaphylaxis; a hazard of multiple cystoscopic examinations under general anaesthesia. *Anaesthesia* **23,** 90—3.

Avery, A. F. and Evans, A. (1973). Reactions to Althesin. *British Journal of Anaesthesia* **45,** 301—3.

Barjenbruch, K. P. and Jones, J. R. (1972). Thiopentone anaphylaxis: a case report. *Anesthesia and Analgesia . . . Current Researches* **51,** 113—16.

Beck, L. (1965). Podiumgesprach uber das Kurznarkotikum Propanidid. In: *Die intravenose Kurznarkose mit dem neuen Phenoxyessigsaurederivat Propanidid (Epontol),* p. 307. Ed. by K. Horatz, R. Frey and M. Zindler. Springer-Verlag, Berlin.

Boytell, K. A. (1976). Anaphylactic reaction to Althesin. *Anaesthesia and Intensive Care* **4,** 362—3.

Bradburn, C. C. (1970). Severe hypotension following induction with propanidid. *British Journal of Anaesthesia* **42,** 362—3.

Brown, T. P. (1975). Thiopentone anaphylaxis — case report. *Anaesthesia and Intensive Care* **3,** 257—9.

Buckett, W. R. (1968). The pharmacology of pancuronium bromide: a new non-depolarising neuromuscular blocking agent. *Irish Journal of Medical Science* **1,** 565—8.

Bussien, R., Rybaric, E. and Thurler, B. (1975). Crise d'asthme après induction avec l'Alfatésine. *Anesthésie, analgésie, réanimation* **32,** 147—8.

Callens, J. and Doutriaux, J. (1976). Deux cas d'allergie sévère en anesthesiologie. *Journal des sciences médicales de Lille* **94,** 293—5.

Carrie, L. E. S. and Buchanan, R. L. (1967). Thiopentone anaphylaxis. *Anaesthesia* **22,** 290—5.

Carson, I. W., Dundee, J. W. and Clarke, R. S. J. (1975). The speed of onset and potency of Althesin. *British Journal of Anaesthesia* **47,** 512—15.

Chan, C. S. and Yeung, M. L. (1972). Anaphylactic reaction to alcuronium. *British Journal of Anaesthesia* **44,** 103—5.

Child, K. J., Currie, J. P., Davis, B., Dodds, M. G., Pearce, D. R. and Twissell, D. J. (1971). The pharmacological properties in animals of CT 1341 — a new steroid anaesthetic agent. *British Journal of Anaesthesia* **43,** 2—13.

Clark, M. M. and Cockburn, H. A. (1971). Anaphylactoid response to thiopentone. *British Journal of Anaesthesia* **43,** 185—9.

Clark, R. M. (1973). Reactions to pancuronium. *British Journal of Anaesthesia* **45,** 997.

Clarke, R. S. J. and Dundee, J. W. (1969). Hypotensive reaction after propanidid and atropine. *British Medical Journal* **4,** 369.

Clarke, R. S. J. and Dundee, J. W. (1970). Toxic effects of intravenous anaesthetics: a comparison of propanidid with thiopentone. In: *Progress in Anaesthesiology*, Proceedings of the 4th World Congress of Anaesthesiologists, Amsterdam, pp. 1189—91. Ed. by T. B. Boulton, R. Bryce-Smith, M. K. Sykes, G. B. Gillett and A. L. Revell. Excerpta Medica, Amsterdam.

Clarke, R. S. J., Dundee, J. W., Barron, D. W., McArdle, L. and Howard, P. J. (1968). Clinical studies of induction agents. XXVI: The relative potencies of thiopentone, methohexitone and propanidid. *British Journal of Anaesthesia* **40,** 593—601.

Clarke, R. S. J., Dundee, J. W. and Carson, I. W. (1972). Some aspects of the clinical pharmacology of Althesin. *Postgraduate Medical Journal* **48,** Suppl. 2., 62—5.

Clarke, R. S. J., Dundee, J. W., Garrett, R. T., McArdle, G. K. and Sutton, J. A. (1975). Adverse reactions to intravenous anaesthetics. A survey of 100 reports. *British Journal of Anaesthesia* **47,** 575-85.

Cole, F. (1968). Sensitivity to thiopental. *Nebraska State Medical Journal* **53,** 478.

Comroe, J. H. and Dripps, R. D. (1946). The histamine-like action of curare and tubocurarine injected intracutaneously and intra-arterially in man. *Anesthesiology* **7,** 260—2.

Crowther, A. N. (1973). Bronchospasm following Althesin anaesthesia. *British Medical Journal* **2,** 775.

Cullen, D. J. (1971). Severe anaphylactic reaction to penicillin during halothane anaesthesia. *British Journal of Anaesthesia* **43,** 410—12.

Currie, T. T. (1970). Anaphylactic manifestations. *Proceedings of the Third Asian Australasian Congress of Anaesthesiology*, pp. 127—31. Butterworth, Sydney.

Currie, T. T., Whittingham, S., Ebringer, A. and Peters, J. S. (1966). Severe anaphylactic reaction to thiopentone: case report. *British Medical Journal* **1,** 1462—3.

Dale, H. H. and Laidlaw, P. P. (1919). Histamine shock. *Journal of Physiology* **52,** 355—90.

Dannemann, H. and Lubke, P. (1970). Komplikationen wahrend Narkosen mit Epontol. *Zeitschrift für praktische Anästhesie und Wiederbelebung* **5,** 273.

Davis, J. (1971). Thiopentone anaphylaxis. Case report. *British Journal of Anaesthesia* **43,** 1191—3.

Davison, T. C. (1943). Intravenous anesthesia in modern surgery (sodium—pentothal—oxygen). *Anesthesia and Analgesia . . . Current Researches* **22,** 52—6.

Doenicke, A. (1975). Propanidid. In: *Recent Progress in Anaesthesiology and Resuscitation,* Proceedings of the IV European Congress of Anaesthesiology, Madrid, 5—11 September 1974, pp. 107—13. Ed. by A. Arias, R. Llaurado, M. A. Nalda and J. N. Lunn. Excerpta Medica, Amsterdam; American Elsevier, New York.

Doenicke, A., Lorenz, W., Beigl, R., Bezecny, H., Uhlig, G., Kalmar, L. Praetorius, B. and Mann, G. (1973). Histamine release after intravenous application of short-acting hypnotics. A comparison of etomidate, Althesin (CT 1341) and propanidid. *British Journal of Anaesthesia* **45,** 1094—104.

Douglas, W. W. (1975). Histamines and antihistamines. In: *The Pharmacological Basis of Therapeutics*, 5th edn. Ed. by L. S. Goodman and S. Gilman. Macmillan, New York.

Driggs, R. L. and O'Day, R. A. (1972). Acute allergic reaction associated with methohexital anesthesia: report of six cases. *Journal of Oral Surgery* **30,** 906—9.

Duhm, B., Maul, W., Medenwald, H., Patzschke, K. and Wegner, L. A. (1965). Tierexperimentelle Untersuchungen mit Propanidid-^{14}C. In: *Die intravenous Kurznarkose mit dem neuen Phenoxyessigsaurederivat propanidid (Epontol)*, pp. 78—88. Ed. by K. Horatz, R. Frey and M. Zindler. Springer-Verlag, Berlin.

Dundee, J. W. (1956). *Thiopentone and Other Thiobarbiturates.* Livingstone, Edinburgh.

Dundee, J. W. (1965). Some effects of premedication on the induction characteristics of intravenous anaesthetics. *Anaesthesia* **20,** 299—314.

Dundee, J. W., Assem, E. S. K., Gaston, J. M., Keilty, S. R., Sutton, J. A., Clarke, R. S. J. and Grainger, D. (1974). Sensitivity to intravenous anaesthetics: a report of three cases. *British Medical Journal* **1,** 63—5.

Dundee, J. W., Fee, J. P. H., McDonald, J. R. and Clarke, R. S. J. (1978). Incidence of atopy and allergy in an anaesthetic patient population. *British Journal of Anaesthesia* **50,** 793—8.

Evans, A. (1971). Reaction to propanidid. *British Journal of Anaesthesia* **43,** 802.

Evans, F. and Gould, J. (1952). Relation between sensitivity to thiopentone, sulphonamides and sunlight. *British Medical Journal* **1,** 417.

Evans, J. M. and Keogh, J. A. M. (1977). Adverse reactions to intravenous anaesthetic induction agents. *British Medical Journal* **2,** 735—6.

Fantera, A. and Maurina, M. (1976). Impiego dell'Althesin dell'introduzione endovenosa dell'anestesia generale e valutazione dei suoi effetti cardicircolatori e respiratori. *Acta anaesthesiologica Italica* **27,** 241—56.

Fee, J. P. H., McDonald, J. R., Dundee, J. W. and Clarke, R. S. J. (1978). Frequency of previous anaesthesia in an anaesthetic population. *British Journal of Anaesthesia* **50,** 917—20.

Fisher, M. M. (1975). Severe histamine mediated reactions to intravenous drugs used in anaesthesia. *Anaesthesia and Intensive Care* **3,** 180—97.

Fisher, M. M. (1976a). Severe histamine mediated reactions to Althesin. *Anaesthesia and Intensive Care* **4,** 33—5.

Fisher, M. M. (1976b). Intradermal testing after severe histamine reactions to intravenous drugs used in anaesthesia. *Anaesthesia and Intensive Care* **4,** 97—104.

Fisher, M. M. (1977a). Hypersensitivity to intravenous anaesthetic agents. *British Journal of Anaesthesia* **49,** 87—8.

Fisher, M. M. (1977b). Intradermal testing after severe reactions to anaesthetic drugs. *Anaesthesia and Intensive Care* **5,** 272.

Fisher, M. M. (1977c). Blood volume replacement in acute anaphylactic cardiovascular collapse related to anaesthesia. *British Journal of Anaesthesia* **49,** 1023—6.

Fisher, T. (1968). Allergies ignored: routine versus thought. *Canadian Medical Association Journal* **99,** 854—5.

Fox, G. S., Wilkinson, R. D. and Rabow, F. I. (1971). Thiopental anaphylaxis: a case and a method for diagnosis. *Anesthesiology* **35,** 655—7.

Gjessing, J. (1969). Hypotension, hypoventilation and delayed recovery after propanidid. *British Journal of Anaesthesia* **41,** 1012.

Gotla, D. W. (1972). Apparent anaphylactic reaction to propanidid. *Anaesthesia* **27,** 16—17.

Grimmeisen, H. (1971). Epontol anaesthesia. *Medizinische Klinik* **66,** 1417.

Guilmet, C. and Joue, P. (1976). Un choc anaphylactique au pentothal à l'induction. *Annales de l'Anesthésiologie Française* **17,** 77—80.

Hainsworth, A. M. and Bingham, W. (1970). An allergic circulatory collapse following the administration of muscle relaxants. *Anaesthesia* **25,** 105—9.

Halpern, S. R., Sellars, W. A., Johnson, R. B., Anderson, D. W., Saperstein, S. and Reisch, J. W. (1973). Development of allergy in infants fed breast, soy or cow milk. *Journal of Allergy and Clinical Immunology* **51,** 139.

Harrfeldt, H. P. (1973). 10 Jahre Kurznarkosen mit Propanidid. In: *Intravenose Narkose mit Propanidid,* pp. 234—42. Ed. by M. Zindler, H. Yamamura and W. Wirth. Springer-Verlag, Berlin.

Hayward, J. R. and Kiester, G. L. (1957). Severe allergic reactions during thiopental sodium anaesthesia. *Journal of Oral Surgery* **15,** 61—3.

Healy, T. E. J. (1973). Bronchospasm following Althesin induction. *Lancet* **ii,** 975.

Heath, M. L. (1973). Bronchospasm in an asthmatic patient following pancuronium. *Anaesthesia* **28,** 437—40.

Hester, J. B. (1973). Reaction to Althesin. *British Journal of Anaesthesia* **45,** 303.

Holmes, R. P., Ross, J. W. and Williams, E. R. (1971). Acute anaphylaxis under anaesthesia. *Anaesthesia* **26,** 363—7.

Horton, J. N. (1973). Adverse reaction to Althesin. *Anaesthesia* **28,** 182—3.

Hunter, A. R. (1943). Dangers of pentothal sodium anaesthesia. *Lancet* **i,** 46—8.

Hurwitz, N. (1969). Predisposing factors in adverse reactions to drugs. *British Medical Journal* **1,** 536—9.

Idsøe, O., Guthe, T., Willcox, R. R. and De Weck, A. L. (1968). Nature and extent of penicillin side-reactions, with particular reference to anaphylactic shock. *Bulletin of the World Health Organization* **38,** 159—88.

Jarvis, C. A. N. (1972). Reaction to propanidid. *British Journal of Anaesthesia* **44,** 989.

Jerums, G., Whittingham, S. and Wilson, P. (1967). Anaphylaxis to suxamethonium. *British Journal of Anaesthesia* **39,** 73.

Johns, G. (1970). Cardiac arrest following induction with propanidid. *British Journal of Anaesthesia* **42,** 74—7.

Katz, A. M., Battit, G. E. and Wilkey, B. R. (1970). An anaphylactoid reaction to penicillin during anesthesia. *Anesthesiology* **32,** 84—6.

Katz, A. M. and Mulligan, P. G. (1972). Bronchospasm induced by suxamethonium. *British Journal of Anaesthesia* **44,** 1097—9.

Kay, B. (1969). Hypotensive reaction after propanidid and atropine. *British Medical Journal* **3,** 413.

Kay, B. (1972). Brietal sodium in children's surgery. In: *Das Ultrakurznarkoticum Methohexital,* pp. 149—58. Ed. by C. Lehmann. Springer-Verlag, Berlin.

Kelly, A. J. and Boman, A. (1973). Anaphylaxis under anaesthesia. *Anaesthesia and Intensive Care* **1,** 322—3.

Kepes, E. R. and Haimovici, H. J. (1959). Allergic reactions to succinylcholine. *Journal of the American Medical Association* **177,** 548.

Kessell, J. and Assem, E. S. K. (1974). An adverse reaction to Althesin. *British Journal of Anaesthesia* **46,** 209.

Kivalo, I., Wist, A. and Mustakallio, M. (1960). Anaphylactic shock in thiopental anesthesia. *Duodecim* **76,** 509—10.

Kruger, H. W. (1970). Anaphylaktischer Schock nach Epontol-Kurznarkosen. *Geburtshilfe und Frauenheilkunde* **30,** 37.

Larard, D. G. (1970). Cardiac arrest following induction with propanidid. *British Journal of Anaesthesia* **42,** 652.

Laxenaire, M. C., Sigiel, M., Moneret-Vautrin, D. A., Moeller, R. and Chastel, A. (1976). Accidents anaphylactoides liés à l'emploi de produits anesthésiques et adjuvants. A propos de 18 cas. *Annales de l'Anesthésiologie Française* **17,** 85—90.

Lopert, H. (1955). Allergic reaction to gallamine triethiodide. *Anaesthesia* **10,** 76.

Lorenz, W., Doenicke, A., Meyer, R., Reimann, J., Kusche, J., Barth, H., Geesing, H., Hutzel, M. and Weissenbacher, B. (1972). Histamine release in man by propanidid and thiopentone: pharmacological effects and clinical consequences. *British Journal of Anaesthesia* **44,** 355—69.

McDowell, S. A. and Clarke, R. S. J. (1969). A clinical comparison of pancuronium with tubocurarine. *Anaesthesia* **24,** 581—90.

Manz, R. and Frank, G. (1969). Zur Frage allergischer Reaktionen nach Epontol. *Anaesthesist* **18,** 223.

Mathieu, A. and Grilliat, J. P. (1976). Correspondence. *British Journal of Anaesthesia* **48,** 49—50.

Mehta, S. (1973). Anaphylactic reaction to Althesin. *Anaesthesia* **28,** 669—72.

Miloschewsky, D. and Cervenkova, M. (1970). Cardiovascular collapse following induction with propanidid. *British Journal of Anaesthesia* **42,** 833.

Moneret-Vautrin, D. A. (1976). Les test préventifs et leurs limites. Conduite à tenir devant le risque d'un accident. *Annales de l'Anesthésiologie Française* **17,** 235—8.

Moneret-Vautrin, D. A., Duc, M. and Sigiel, M. (1976). Etude de différents facteurs de risque du déclenchement d'accidents aux anesthésique et myorelaxants. *Annales de l'Anesthésiologie Française* **17,** 165—74.

Mongar, J. L. and Schild, H. O. (1962). Cellular mechanisms in anaphylaxis. *Physiological Reviews* **42,** 226—70.

Monteil, A., Navarrot, P., Kiencen, J. and Du Cailar, J. (1976). A propos de deux observations de reaction de type anaphylactique à l'alfadione (Alfatesin-Althesin CT 1341). *Annales de l'Anesthésiologie Française* **17,** 71—6.

Notcutt, W. G. (1973). Adverse reaction to Althesin. *Anaesthesia* **28,** 673—4.

Pepys, J. (1973). Types of allergic reaction. In: *Clinical Immunology—Allergy in Paediatric Medicine,* vol. 1, p. 4. Ed. by J. Brostoff. Blackwell Scientific Publications, Oxford.

Radnay, P. (1965). Allergic and anaphylactic reactions, decrease in blood pressure. In: *Intravenous anaesthesia for outpatients,* Ed. by M. Zindler. *Acta anaesthesiologica Scandinavica* Suppl. 17, 80.

Rawicz, M., Rondio, Z. and Cwizewicz-Adamska, J. (1976). Anaphylactic shock following Althesin. A case report. *Anaesthesia, Resuscitation and Intensive Therapy* **4,** 65—9.

Reichert, E. F. and Bassett, P. A. (1972). A rare allergic reaction to sodium methohexital. *Journal of Oral Surgery* **30,** 910.

Ring, J. and Messmer, K. (1977). Incidence and severity of anaphylactoid reactions to colloid volume substitutes. *Lancet* **i,** 466—9.

Rozenkranz, I. (1972). Cardiovascular collapse after propanidid. *British Journal of Anaesthesia* **44,** 1332.

Saint-Maurice, C., Daihle-Dupont, D., Roche, M., Fulin, M. and Viallard, C. (1976). Deux cas de réactions de type anaphylactique en rapport avec l'anesthésie. *Annales de l'Anesthésiologie Française* **17,** 81—4.

Salem, M. R., Kim, Y. and El Etr, A. A. (1968). Histamine release following intravenous injection of *d*-tubocurarine. *Anesthesiology* **29,** 380—2.

Samuel, I. O. and Dundee, J. W. (1973). Clinical studies of induction agents. XLII: Influence of injection rate and dosage on the induction complications with Althesin. *British Journal of Anaesthesia* **45,** 1215—16.

Sargent, N. W. (1971). Anaphylactoid reaction to thiopentone. *British Journal of Anaesthesia* **43,** 591.

Savege, T. M., Foley, E. I. and Simpson, B. R. (1973). Some cardio-respiratory effects of Cremophor EL in man. *British Journal of Anaesthesia* **45,** 515—17.

Scholtan, E. and Lie, S. Y. (1966). Kolloid-chemische Eigenschaften eines neuen Kurznarkoticums. *Arzneimittel-Forschung* **16,** 679—91.

Shafto, C. E. (1969). Continuous intravenous anaesthesia for paediatric dentistry. *British Journal of Anaesthesia* **41,** 407—16.

Shaw, H. (1974). Anaesthetic complications. *New Zealand Society of Anaesthetists' Newsletter* **21,** 144.

Sneddon, I. B. and Glew, R. C. (1973). Contact dermatitis due to propanidid in an anaesthetist. *Practitioner* **211,** 321—3.

Soga, D., Beer, R., Bader, B., Andrae, J. and Gotz, E. (1973). Die Beeinflussung der linksventrikularen Myokardkontraktilitat und Haemodynamik durch Propanidid beim Menschen. In: *Intravenous Narkose mit Propanidid,* pp. 78—87. Ed. by M. Zindler, H. Yamamura and W. Wirth. Springer-Verlag, Berlin.

Spreadbury, T. H. and Marrett, H. R. (1971). Cardiovascular collapse after propanidid. *British Journal of Anaesthesia* **43,** 925.

Spruill, F. G., Minette, L. J. and Sturner, W. Q. (1974). Two surgical deaths associated with cephalothin. *Journal of the American Medical Association* **229,** 440—1.

Steel, G. C. (1976). Reaction to Althesin. *British Journal of Anaesthesia* **48,** 50.

Stieglitz, P., Jacquot, C. and Riondel, J. P. (1976). Accidents d'histamino-libération per-anesthésique. *Annales de l'Anesthésiologie Française* **17,** 91—4.

Stovner, J. and Endresen, R. (1971). Repeated propanidid in cancer. *British Journal of Anaesthesia* **43,** 207—8.

Strunk, H. A. (1962). Reaction to thiopental. *Anesthesiology* **23,** 271.

Sutton, J. A. (1976). Mechanism of a reaction to Althesin. *British Journal of Anaesthesia* **48,** 711—12.

Thompson, D. S., Eason, C. N. and Flacke, J. E. (1973). Thiamylal anaphylaxis. *Anesthesiology* **39,** 556—8.

Thornton, H. L. (1971). Apparent anaphylactic reaction to propanidid. *Anaesthesia* **26,** 490—3.

Turner, K. J., Keep, V. R. and Bartholomaeus, N. (1972). Anaphylaxis induced by propanidid and atropine. *British Journal of Anaesthesia* **44,** 211.

Tweedie, D. G. and Ordish, P. M. (1974). Reactions to intravenous agents (Althesin and pancuronium). *British Journal of Anaesthesia* **46,** 244.

Unsworth, I. P. (1972). Thiopentone anaphylaxis. *Anaesthesia and Intensive Care* **1,** 79—80.

Velazquez, J. L. and Gold, M. I. (1975). Anaphylactic reaction to cephalothin during anesthesia. *Anesthesiology* **43,** 476—8.

Vervloet, D., Arnaud, A., Vellieux, P., Kaplanski, S. and Charpin, J. (1977). Accident de type anaphylactique imputables aux myorelaxants au cours de l'anesthésie général. Etude clinique et biologique. *Nouvelle Presse Medicale* **6,** 725—8.

Vignon, H., Gay, R. and Laxenaire, M. C. (1976). Observations cliniques d'accidents anaphylactoides per et post anesthésiques. Résultat d'enquêtes a posteriori. *Annales de l'Anesthésiologie Française* **17,** 117—21.

Walmsley, D. A. (1959). Sensitivity reaction to gallamine triethiodide. *Lancet* **ii,** 237—8.

Watkins, J., Clark, A., Appleyard, T. N. and Padfield, A. (1976a). Immune-mediated reactions to Althesin (alphaxalone). *British Journal of Anaesthesia* **48,** 881—6.

Watkins, J., Udnoon, S., Appleyard, T. N. and Thornton, J. A. (1976b). Identification and quantitation of hypersensitivity reactions to intravenous anaesthetic agents. *British Journal of Anaesthesia* **48,** 457—61.

Watkins, J., Udnoon, S. and Taussig, P. (1978). In: *Adverse Response to Intravenous Drugs.* Ed. by J. Watkins and A. M. Ward. Academic Press, London.

Watt, J. M. (1975). Anaphylactic reactions after use of CT 1341 (Althesin). *British Medical Journal* **3,** 205—6.

Wedley, J. R. (1973). Thiopentone-induced bronchospasm. *Anaesthesia* **28,** 318—19.

Werner, M. and Wolff, E. (1970). Klinisch-experimentelle Untersuchungen zur Frage de Propanidid-Allergie. In: *Intravenose Narkose mit Propanidid*, p. 217. Ed. by M. Zindler, H. Yamamura and W. Wirth. Springer-Verlag, Berlin.

Westgate, H. D., Schultz, E. A. and Van Bergen, F. H. (1961). Urticaria and angioneurotic edema following *d*-tubocurarine administration. *Anesthesiology* **22,** 286.

Wyatt, R. and Watkins, J. (1975). Reaction to methohexitone. *British Journal of Anaesthesia* **47,** 1119—20.

Zindler, M. (1965). Allergic and anaphylactic reactions, decrease in blood pressure. In: *Intravenous anaesthesia for ourpatients.* Edited by M. Zindler. *Acta anaesthesiologica Scandinavica* Suppl. 17, 79—80.

Zindler, M. (1975). Propanidid (Epontol): reappraisal of its present position. In: *Recent Progress in Anaesthesiology and Resuscitation*, Proceedings of the IV European Congress of Anaesthesiology, Madrid, 5—11 September 1974, pp. 114—17. Ed. by A. Arias, R. Llaurado, M. A. Nalda and J. N. Lunn. Excerpta Medica, Amsterdam; American Elsevier, New York.

9

Balanced techniques

It is not proposed to devote a specific chapter to the topic of neurolept anaesthesia (or analgesia) as this is simply a terminology for a balanced technique of anaesthesia which includes a potent analgesic and a hypnotic. Basically it is little different from the technique of 'artificial hibernation' popularized by Laborit and Huguenard in the mid-1950s. We now have newer and shorter-acting drugs which are possibly less toxic than the original pethidine—chlorpromazine—promethazine sequence, but basically the concept remains unchanged. Neurolept techniques (NLA) vary from hospital to hospital and are adequately described in most standard texts and in the fall 1973 issue of *International Anesthesiology Clinics* (Oyama, 1973). Rather than covering old ground, attention in this chapter is focused on some specific topics including the drugs used in NLA, some advantages recently claimed for the technique, the new analgesic buprenorphine and a personal assessment of balanced techniques.

Definitions and terminology

The following is taken from Foldes (1973) who contributed the chapter on NLA for general surgery in the publication referred to above. It helps to clarify the terminology as regards neurolept techniques.

> 'The term *neuroleptanalgesia* was first proposed by de Castro and Mundeleer (1959) to describe a state of indifference and immobilization, termed *mineralization* and produced by the combined administration of the neuroleptic (ataractic) drug, haloperidol (Haldol, Serenace), and the narcotic analgesic (narcotic), phenoperidine (Operidine). Subsequently the technique underwent several modifications by other investigators who, instead of phenoperidine, used other narcotics and short-acting barbiturates for induction of anesthesia and nitrous oxide-oxygen to maintain anesthesia. After 1963, when droperidol (Droleptan, Inapsine) and fentanyl lactate (Sublimaze) were made available (Janssen *et al.*, 1963), these compounds became the most widely used ataractic and narcotic components of neuroleptanalgesia.
>
> 'Patients who receive nitrous oxide—oxygen in addition to droperidol and fentanyl not only become analgesic and sedated but also lose consciousness or, in other words, become anesthetized. The term *neuroleptanesthesia* was proposed (Foldes *et al.*, 1966) to characterize the state of these patients. It was suggested that the term *neuroleptanalgesia* be restricted to those patients who under the influence of neuroleptic

> and narcotic drugs become analgesic, deeply sedated and partly or wholly amnesic, but are capable of obeying commands and answering simple questions during surgery.
>
> 'Neuroleptanesthesia induced with a fixed 50:1 mixture of droperidol and fentanyl citrate (Innovar, Thalamonal) and nitrous oxide—oxygen rapidly became a widely used anesthetic technique. It was reported that neuroleptanesthesia caused little or no impairment of the circulatory hemostasis in poor risk (Corssen, Domino and Sweet, 1964) and geriatric (Aubry *et al.*, 1965) patients and had a beneficial effect in hemorrhagic or other types of hypovolemic shock (Corssen, Domino and Sweet, 1964). It was also observed that patients usually regained consciousness promptly after discontinuation of anesthesia (Holderness, Chase and Dripps, 1963) but remained tranquil and cooperative postoperatively, and that the incidence of nausea and emesis (Crossen, Domino and Sweet, 1964; Holderness, Chase and Dripps, 1963) was diminished and narcotic requirements were reduced (Corssen, Domino and Sweet, 1964).

This quotation may seem superfluous to some but there is much confusion on terminology and the relationship of NLA to other drugs. One was surprised to find droperidol classed as an intravenous induction agents in a recent non-anaesthetic publication. More surprising was its listing under 'Anesthetics, intravenous' in the 1977 volume 46 index of *Anesthesiology*. While it is a constituent of one form of NLA, it should never be looked on as an induction agent (see Chapter 1).

'Pentazepam' is the name given by Aldrete and his colleagues (1971) to a 3:1 mixture of pentazocine and diazepam — undoubtedly a variation of the original NLA. In this case they combined it with nitrous oxide—oxygen and produced very satisfactory anaesthesia. Perhaps we may next hear of 'Diazocine'!

Drugs

The drugs used in NLA have varied over the years and the relative merits of some of these are reviewed below: the sedative part of the mixture is considered first, followed by the analgesic component. The relative value of some of the mixtures is also discussed. The drugs fall into two main groups — sedative—tranquillizers and potent analgesics. Some of the former are discussed elsewhere and repetition is kept to a minimum.

Sedative—tranquillizers

Those used in NLA fall into three chemical groups:

1. Phenothiazines: chlorpromazine, promethazine, etc.
2. Butyrophenones: haloperidol, droperidol.
3. Benzodiazepines: diazepam and similar drugs.

The first two groups, in addition to their sedative and tranquillizing action, have marked anti-emetic properties and will counteract the tendency of the potent narcotics to produce nausea and vomiting. The phenothiazines are not discussed here. Neither is haloperidol which in clinical doses is followed by too high an incidence of extrapyramidal effects to make it acceptable for NLA.

Droperidol

This must be one of the most controversial drugs used in anaesthetic practice. It can be given intravenously and intramuscularly, and has definite sedative and tranquillizing effects. It is two to three minutes before sedation occurs following intravenous injection and its action lasts for several hours. It has no analgesic action of its own, nor does it potentiate the action of potent narcotics although it does prolong their action.

Droperidol is claimed to produce a state of indifference to one's surroundings, with patients being placid and drowsy, although easily rousable. Paradoxically, although they may appear to be placid, many patients are more apprehensive than before injection and some exhibit hypertonus and motor restlessness (dyskinesia) which can be very unpleasant. As a group, the butyrophenones can produce catalepsy with spontaneous movement and other evidence of extrapyramidal activity. Oculogyric crises can occur up to four hours after its administration. All the excitatory central nervous system effects are reduced in incidence and severity when droperidol is given with an opiate, and the author feels strongly that it should never be given alone to a conscious patient.

One real advantage of droperidol is its mild alpha-adrenergic blocking action, which has been demonstrated in animals (Muldoon *et al.*, 1977) and man (Whitwam and Russell, 1971). This produces a slight fall in blood pressure and postural hypotension which can facilitate the production of a bloodless operative field. It is also useful to counteract harmful vasoconstriction in 'shock' states but one must be careful to avoid its use in the presence of hypovolaemia.

Diazepam

This has recently been used in NLA techniques in combination with potent analgesics. Its sedative and amnesic actions have already been reviewed in Chapter 7. One cannot readily equate scientifically its sedative—tranquillizing action with that of droperidol; in practice it appears to be more soporific and probably longer acting. It is virtually free from the excitatory and cataleptic effects of the butyrophenones.

In contrast with droperidol (and hydroxyzine) which Cottrell, Wolfson and Siker (1976) found caused increased airway resistance, diazepam produced no effects on pulmonary compliance in volunteers. The drugs were given by intramuscular injection in doses of 0.1 mg·kg^{-1} diazepam and 0.07 mg·kg^{-1} droperidol, which would appear to be equipotent as tranquillizers. Because of unpleasant side effects (restlessness and irritability), there were only four subjects in the droperidol study.

Analgesics

Virtually every available analgesic has been used in NLA but discussion here is limited to a few of these drugs.

Dextromoramide. The first opiate to be used in NLA, this methadone derivative is a long-acting analgesic. It has some popularity in the relief of postoperative and chronic pain (given orally or intramuscularly) but is rarely used intravenously during anaesthesia.

Pethidine. This was the first analgesic to be used widely during anaesthesia. It was the analgesic component of the lytic cocktail and is sometimes given with droperidol to lessen its emetic effects. It is a potentially toxic drug which may release histamine on intravenous injection and cause sudden hypotension; its popularity as an intravenous analgesic may be due to its rapid onset and brevity of action. These features have certainly contributed to its safe use in obstetrics.

Phenoperidine. A newer derivative of the pethidine series, this has a similar time course of events to the parent compound. It is relatively free from the hypotensive action of pethidine but causes profound respiratory depression in effective doses.

Fentanyl. This is a relatively short-acting analgesic with actions qualitatively similar to those of morphine or pethidine. It is about 100 times more potent than morphine and approximately equianalgesic doses are 0.1 mg fentanyl, 10 mg morphine and 75 mg pethidine. Its introduction into NLA may have resulted from its rapid onset and brevity of action but the fact that it was marketed by the same pharmaceutical companies as droperidol obviously played a part. It has a wide safety margin and recent studies have again confirmed cardiovascular stability even after larger doses (Stoelting *et al.*, 1975; Lui *et al.*, 1976). The addition of nitrous oxide—oxygen does appear to reduce its safety.

On the debit side, fentanyl is not infrequently followed by ventilatory difficulties caused by rigidity of the respiratory muscles. This creates no difficulty in the relaxed unconscious patient but can cause problems when it is given for analgesia without loss of consciousness. A report of the personal experience of a patient who developed such difficulties and who was eventually given suxamethonium has lessened the enthusiasm of the author for its use as an intravenous analgesic. Recent reports draw attention to the possibility of a delayed onset of respiratory depression in the post-operative period after large doses of fentanyl (Adams and Pybus, 1978) but it is difficult to be sure whether this would not have happened with any narcotic analgesic. Fentanyl-induced respiratory depression quickly responds to adequate doses of naloxone (Drummond, Davie and Scott, 1977).

Pentazocine. Theoretically, this mixed opiate antagonist—agonist has much to recommend it as a supplement to general anaesthesia and as part of an NLA regimen. It appears to cause less respiratory and cardiovascular depression than other potent analgesics and in effective doses it is less soporific. High doses may cause hallucinations and other unpleasant effects but these are prevented by its combination with diazepam.

For an up-to-date survey of the actions of pentazocine, the reviews by Brogden, Speight and Avery (1973) and the editorial by Payne (1973) are recommended.

Morphine: With the advent of cardiac surgery and the feasibility, and even desirability, of prolonged postoperative ventilation, morphine is finding a place as a supplement to orthodox anaesthesia, as part of a NLA technique or as the sole agent (see Chapter 10). Its therapeutic action lasts as long as that of diazepam and droperidol, which will minimize its emetic and dysphoric actions.

Mixtures

The premixed 50:1 droperidol–fentanyl is the most popular NLA combination, and is widely used as a premedicant and sometimes for the induction and/or maintenance of anaesthesia. The use of fixed mixtures has justifiably been criticized, and in the case of Innovar/Thalamonal there is the additional criticism of a short-acting narcotic being combined with a long-acting neuroplegic. The combination becomes more acceptable if it is reserved for premedication or the induction period and fentanyl alone is used for supplementation during anaesthesia. The intermittent use of the mixture can lead to the unpleasant side effects of droperidol appearing in the postoperative period.

Because of their similar duration of action, phenoperidine and droperidol can be used together. This mixture avoids the risk of respiratory complications of fentanyl, but will cause respiratory depression. The author and colleagues (Stevenson *et al.*, 1972) prefer a mixture containing 2 mg phenoperidine with 5—10 mg droperidol (depending on the weight and physical condition of the patient) and find it very satisfactory for endoscopic procedures. If the dose of droperidol is restricted, it will be less soporific than a diazepam—phenoperidine combination, and if respiratory depression occurs patients will take deep breaths when requested.

The lesser soporific action of pentazocine, as compared with other opiates, allows the use of the more soporific diazepam, which has useful properties. Its use in the mixture known as 'Pentazepam' has already been mentioned.

An infusion containing 90 mg pentazocine and 30 mg diazepam in 250 ml 5 per cent dextrose in water has been used in unpremedicated patients for laporoscopic sterilization (Aldrete *et al.*, 1976). Respiration was spontaneous throughout with 3 l·min^{-1} nasal oxygen, and the changes in arterial blood gases were minimal. This combination would seem to have much to recommend it. Both drugs have a similar duration of action, neither causes marked respiratory depression and the tranquillizers would, it is hoped, control the unpleasant psychic effects of large doses of the opiate. Prolonged recovery would be expected to be the major problem with the large doses used, but this has not been commented upon in reports (Guillen and Aldrete, 1970; Aldrete, 1971).

If flunitrazepam were available as an intravenous preparation it would be preferred to diazepam in this situation.

Buprenorphine

The new synthetic opiate analgesic of the oripavine series of compounds has recently been introduced into clinical practice. Like pentazocine, it is a partial agonist with both agonist and antagonist effects and it will precipitate abstinence (withdrawal) symptoms in morphine-dependent subjects. However, these do not occur with the chronic use of buprenorphine or when treated patients are given naloxone, a narcotic antagonist. It is claimed from studies on animals and humans that this analgesic has a low addiction potential.

Buprenorphine is available in an aqueous solution containing 0.3 mg·ml^{-1} which can be administered both intramuscularly and intravenously. On its initial release it was recommended as a strong analgesic for use in moderate and severe pain in postoperative patients, postmyocardial infarction and terminal malignancy. In addition to these indications, it is being used as an intravenous supplement during general anaesthesia and for the production of long-term analgesia in an intensive care situation. For this reason some of its properties are reviewed in this chapter. For a more detailed description the publication of Harcus, Smith and Whittle (1977) should be consulted.

When given intramuscularly, 4–8 μg·kg^{-1} buprenorphine is an effective analgesic for adults (Hovell, 1977). Analgesia from 4 μg·kg^{-1} can last for at least 6 hours. A dose of 0.4 mg was found by Hovell and Ward (1977) to produce better pain relief than 10 mg morphine.

In another study, Downing, Leary and White (1977) recorded 7–8 hours' analgesia from 0.6 mg buprenorphine as compared with 3–4 hours with 15 mg morphine. When given intravenously, the onset of action occurs within 15 minutes (McQuillan, 1976) while other studies suggest that it is slightly slower acting than morphine. Our own clinical experience has shown buprenorphine to be a very potent long-lasting analgesic with a slightly slower onset of action than morphine and a considerably slower onset than pethidine.

Most reports show that the cardiovascular and respiratory effects of buprenorphine are similar to those of equivalent doses of morphine. However, when given intravenously during anaesthesia, prolonged respiratory depression has occurred in the postoperative period in adults given 0.6 mg buprenorphine. This only became marked when patients had left the operating theatre and when they were undisturbed in bed. A similar state has been reported after fentanyl but in the experience of the author and colleagues this is more frequent after buprenorphine — it seems to occur so frequently that one hesitates to use doses as high as 0.6 mg during anaesthesia in curarized patients. The situation does not appear to be of such serious import in spontaneously breathing patients. It is important to note that, in normal adult doses, naloxone produces a very brief, incomplete reversal of the respiratory effects of buprenorphine (Orwin, 1977) while doxapram is more effective in this respect. Since this respiratory stimulant — unlike the antagonist naloxone — does not abolish analgesia, it is recommended that an infusion of 100 mg doxapram in 500 ml dextrose or salt solution be given postoperatively to patients receiving this narcotic, the drip rate being adjusted to maintain adequate respiratory exchange.

Although it does not appear to produce the severe hallucinogenic effects of large doses of pentazocine, buprenorphine is not entirely free from this unpleasant complication. Marked emotional upset has been observed after 0.6 mg given postoperatively.

Neither of these complications need distract from the very real beneficial effects of buprenorphine. They must, however, be taken as an indication for caution lest abuse of the drug causes it to fall into disrepute.

The use of buprenorphine in patients receiving artificial ventilation seems worthy of exploration — here complete analgesia could be achieved without fear of respiratory depression. Its combination with lorazepam would seem appropriate as these two long-acting drugs would give a prolonged period of analgesia and amnesia. Furthermore, the benzodiazepines may reduce the danger of psychotic sequelae with this drug, as they do with ketamine.

Cerebral blood flow

One of the advantages claimed for NLA is a reduction in cerebral blood flow with a corresponding decrease in cerebral oxygen consumption. Early animal studies yielded conflicting results with droperidol—fentanyl: an increase in cats (Nilsson and Ingvar, 1966) and a decrease in dogs (Michenfelder and Theye, 1971). Barker and his colleagues (1968) found no significant effect from the same combination in man. However, Vernhiet *et al.* (1978) found a significant reduction (34 per cent) in cerebral blood flow with a diazepam—fentanyl mixture, with a decrease in $CMRO_2$ of a similar degree. This means that, although good operating conditions will be produced by this combination, there will be no specific protection of the brain against hypoxia.

USELA

This interesting abbreviation is for Undesirable Side Effects of Light Anaesthesia (Abouleish and Taylor, 1976), which include awareness, pain and/or unpleasant dreams. The problems of awareness during operation, particularly in operative obstetrics, have already been discussed in Chapter 7, while unpleasant dreams are mentioned in Chapter 5.

Abouleish and Taylor (1976) recommend that a morphine—diazepam mixture be injected intravenously following delivery of the baby using doses of 0.2 $mg{\cdot}kg^{-1}$ morphine and 0.1 $mg{\cdot}kg^{-1}$ diazepam. This resulted in a 3.4 per cent incidence of recall and unpleasant dreams, and they claim that this mixture produces retrograde amnesia. However, these authors do not give their own incidence of USELA in a 'control' series, nor do they produce any evidence for retrograde amnesia. Rather, a comparison is made with the published results of the series of Wilson and Turner (1969). One does not doubt that a morphine—diazepam mixture will result in a low incidence of USELA — in fact, this applies to any form of adequately balanced general anaesthesia.

Phaeochromocytoma — a contraindication?

In view of the fact that droperidol antagonizes the pressor effects of adrenaline and noradrenaline (Yelnosky, Katz and Diertrich, 1964; Whitwam and Russell, 1971) and prevents catecholamine-induced dysrhythmias in man (Long, Dripps and Price, 1967), it is not surprising that it has been given to patients undergoing operations for phaeochromocytoma. In this situation the mild alpha-adrenergic blocking effect of droperidol has proved very beneficial (Clarke, Tobias and Challen, 1972; Ogawa and Fujita, 1972). However, two reports from Japan described the occurrence of extreme hypertension resulting from the NLA (Morikawa *et al.*, 1972; Yusa, 1973). This responded readily to alpha-adrenergic blockers; however its mechanism is uncertain.

A recent report, again from Japan (Sumikawa and Amakata, 1977), describes another case in which the restlessness following droperidol was accompanied by a rise in pressure to 230/160. When given during the operation, the blood pressure again rose to 205/100 within a minute. Perhaps there may be some significance in the fact that all these reports of droperidol-induced hypertension are from one country. However, attention is drawn to the fact that this theoretically desirable form of anaesthesia should not be used in patients undergoing operation for phaeochromocytoma, particularly if droperidol is included in the mixture. A theoretical consideration might well suggest that droperidol—fentanyl (Thalamonal) would be a good premedicant for such cases, whereas in practice it should be avoided.

Personal assessment

As mentioned previously, there is no mystique about NLA — it is simply a scientific combination of a potent analgesic, perhaps given in apnoeic doses, with a sedative—tranquillizer which preferably has an anti-emetic and/or amnesic action. In a comment on the study of 'Memory under diazepam—morphine neuroleptanestheisa in male surgical patients' (Eisenberg, Taub and Burana, 1974) the reviewer (Larcom, 1975) expresses views which are in accord with those of the author:

> 'The use of drugs similar to droperidol and fentanyl as supplements to a nitrous oxide—relaxant technique certainly is clinically sound. There is no magic about the above combination. In fact, sound management of balanced anesthesia requires flexibility of agents tailored to the duration and type of surgery, i.e. anticipation of a short procedure would dictate a short acting narcotic like fentanyl. The paired drugs in the 'Innovar' preparation has frequently been criticized. The use of a short acting narcotic appears sound, but why pair it with a long acting tranquillizer with alpha blocking qualities? This may leave the postoperative patient at risk to postural hypotension and prolonged sedation without analgesia.
>
> 'It has been demonstrated that large doses of morphine (1 to 3 mg per kg) are not anesthetic or amnesic. Diazepam is a good amnesic and is associated with little cardiovascular and respiratory depression while producing the desired clinical result. The combination of diazepam—morphine neuroleptanesthesia is clinically sound for procedures over 60 minutes in duration, or with titrated doses.'

References

Abouleish, E. and Taylor, F. H. (1976). Effect of morphine—diazepam on signs of anesthesia, awareness and dreams of patients under N_2O for cesarean section. *Anesthesia and Analgesia . . . Current Researches* **55,** 702—5.

Adams, A. P. and Pybus, D. A. (1978). Delayed respiratory depression after use of fentanyl during anaesthesia. *British Medical Journal* **1,** 278—9.

Aldrete, J. A. (1971). Respiratory changes during laryngoscopy: influence of the anesthetic technique. *ORL Digest* **22,** 29—35.

Aldrete, J. A., Clapp, H. W., Fishman, J. and O'Higgins, J. W. (1971). 'Pentazepam' a supplementary agent. *Anesthesia and Analgesia . . . Current Researches* **50,** 498—504.

Aldrete, J. A., Tan, S. T., Carrow, D. J. and Watts, M. K. (1976). 'Pentazepam' (pentazocine + diazepam) supplementing local analgesia for laparoscopic sterilization. *Anesthesia and Analgesia . . . Current Researches* **55,** 177—81.

Aubry, U., Carignan, G., Charette, D., Kerri-Szanto, M. and Lavalee, J. P. (1965). Neuroleptanalgesia with fentanyl—droperidol. An appreciation based on more than 1,000 anaesthetics for major surgery. *Canadian Anaesthetists' Society Journal* **13,** 263.

Barker, J., Harper, A. M., McDowall, D. G., Fitch, W. and Jennett, W. B. (1968). Cerebral blood flow, cerebrospinal fluid pressure and EEG activity during neuroleptanalgesia induced with dehydrobenzperidol and phenoperidol. *British Journal of Anaesthesia* **40,** 143—4.

Brogden, R. N., Speight, T. M. and Avery, G. S. (1973). Pentazocine: a review of its pharmacological properties, therapeutic efficacy and dependence liability. *Drugs* **5,** 6—91.

Clarke, A. D., Tobias, M. A. and Challen, P. D. (1972). The use of neuroleptanalgesia during surgery for phaeochromocytoma. Report of two cases. *British Journal of Anaesthesia* **44,** 1093—6.

Corssen, G., Domino, E. F. and Sweet, R. B. (1964). Neuroleptanalgesia and anesthesia. *Anesthesia and Analgesia . . . Current Researches* **43,** 748—62.

Cottrell, J. E., Wolfson, B. and Siker, E. S. (1976). Changes in airway resistance following droperidol, hydroxyzine and diazepam in normal volunteers. *Anesthesia and Analgesia . . . Current Researches* **55,** 18—21.

de Castro, G. and Mundeleer, P. (1959). Anesthesie sans sommeil 'La neuroleptanalgesie'. *Acta chirurgica Belgica* **58,** 689.

Downing, J. W., Leary, W. P. and White, E. S. (1977). Buprenorphine: a new potent long-acting synthetic analgesic. Comparison with morphine. *British Journal of Anaesthesia* **49,** 251—5.

Drummond, G. B., Davie, I. T. and Scott, D. B. (1977). Naloxone: dose-dependent antagonism of respiratory depression by fentanyl in anaesthetised patients. *British Journal of Anaesthesia* **49,** 151—4.

Eisenberg, L., Taub, H. A. and Burana, A. (1974). Memory under diazepam—morphine neuroleptanesthesia in male surgical patients. *Anesthesia and Analgesia . . . Current Researches* **53,** 488—94.

Foldes, F. F. (1973). Neuroleptanesthesia for general surgery. In: *Neuroleptanesthesia* Ed. by T. Oyama. *International Anesthesiology Clinics* **11,** 1—35. Little, Brown, Boston.

Foldes, F. F., Kepes, E. R., Kronfeld, P. P. and Shiffman, H. P. (1966). A rational approach to neuroleptanesthesia. *Anesthesia and Analgesia . . . Current Researches* **45,** 642.

Guillen, J. and Aldrete, J. A. (1970). Anesthetic factors influencing morbidity and mortality of elderly patients undergoing inguinal herniorrhapy. *American Journal of Surgery* **120,** 760—3.

Harcus, A. W., Smith, R. B. and Whittle, B. A. (Eds) (1977). *Pain: New Perspectives in Measurement and Management.* Churchill Livingstone, Edinburgh and London.

Holderness, M. C., Chase, P. E. and Dripps, R. D. (1963). A narcotic analgesic and a butyrophenone with nitrous oxide for general anesthesia. *Anesthesiology* **24,** 336.

Hovell, B. C. (1977). Comparison of buprenorphine, pethidine and pentazocine for the relief of pain after operation. *British Journal of Anaesthesia* **49,** 913—16.

Hovell, B. C. and Ward, A. E. (1977). Pain relief in the postoperative period: a comparative trial of morphine and a new analgesic buprenorphine. *Journal of International Medical Research* **5,** 417—21.

Janssen, P. A. J., Niemegeers, C. J. E., Schellekens, K. H. I., Verbruggen, F. J. and Van Nueten, J. M. (1963). The pharmacology of dehydrobenzperidol, a new potent and short acting neuroleptic agent chemically related to haloperidol. *Arzneimittel-Forschung* **13,** 205—11.

Laborit, H. and Huguenard, P. (1954). *Pratique de l'hibernothérapie en chirurgie et en médecine.* Masson, Paris.

Larcom, G. D. Jr. (1975). Review of Eisenberg, L., Taub, H. A. and Burana, A. (1974), Anesthesia and Analgesia . . . Current Researches **53,** 488—94. *Survey of Anesthesiology* **19,** 258.

Long, G., Dripps, R. D. and Price, H. L. (1967). Measurement of anti-arrhythmic potency of drugs in man: effects of dehydrobenzperidol. *Anesthesiology* **28,** 318.

Lui, W.-S., Bidwai, A. V., Stanley, T. H. and Isern-Amaral, J. (1976). Cardiovascular dynamics after large doses of fentanyl and fentanyl plus N_2O in the dog. *Anesthesia and Analgesia . . . Current Researches* **55,** 168—72.

McQuillan, D. A. (1976). Buprenorphine pain relief following Caesarean section. *Abstract 205,* Sixth World Congress of Anesthesiology. Excerpta Medica, Amsterdam.

Michenfelder, J. D. and Theye, R. A. (1971). Effects of fentanyl, droperidol and Innovar on canine cerebral metabolism and blood flow. *British Journal of Anaesthesia* **41,** 554.

Morikawa, S., Hikita, K., Arukawa, S. and Iwai, S. (1972). α-Blocking and anti-arrhythmic effect of droperidol. *Japanese Journal of Anaesthesia* **21,** 1268—74.

Muldoon, S. M., Janssens, W. J., Verbeuren, T. J. and Vanhoutte, P. M. (1977). Alpha-adrenergic blocking properties of droperidol on isolated blood vessels of the dog. *British Journal of Anaesthesia* **49,** 211—16.

Nilsson, E. and Ingvar, D. H. (1966). Cerebral blood flow during neuroleptanalgesia in cats. *Acta anaesthesiologica Scandinavica* **10,** 47.

Ogawa, R. and Fujita, A. (1972). Neuroleptanesthesia for the surgery of pheochromocytoma. *Japanese Journal of Anesthesia* **21,** 174—8.

Orwin, J. M. (1977). The effect of doxapram on buprenorphine-induced respiratory depression. *Acta anesthesiologica Belgica* **28,** 93—106.

Oyama, T. (Ed.) (1973). *Neuroleptanesthesia. International Anesthesiology Clinics* **11,** No. 3. Little, Brown, Boston.

Payne, J. P. (1973). The clinical pharmacology of pentazocine. *Drugs* **5,** 1—5.

Stevenson, H. M., Pandit, S. K., Dundee, J. W., McDowell, S. and Morrison, J. D. (1972). Experiences with a technique of neurolept-analgesia for bronchography. *Thorax* **27,** 334—7.

Stoelting, R. K., Gibbs, P. S., Creasser, C. W. and Peterson, C. (1975). Hemodynamic and ventilatory responses to fentanyl, fentanyl—droperidol and nitrous oxide in patients with acquired valvular heart disease. *Anesthesiology* **42,** 319—24.

Sumikawa, K. and Amakata, Y. (1977). The pressor effect of droperidol on a patient with phaeochromocytoma. *Anesthesiology* **46,** 359—61.

Vernhiet, J., Renou, A. M., Orgogozo, J. M., Constant, P. and Caille, J. M. (1978). Effects of a diazepam—fentanyl mixture on cerebral blood flow and oxygen consumption in man. *British Journal of Anaesthesia* **50,** 165—9.

Whitwam, J. G. and Russell, W. J. (1971). The acute cardiovascular changes and adrenergic blockade by droperidol in man. *British Journal of Anaesthesia* **43,** 581—91.

Wilson, J. and Turner, D. J. (1969). Awareness during Caesarean section under general anaesthesia. *British Medical Journal* **1,** 280.

Yelnosky, J., Katz, R. and Diertrich, E. V. (1964). A study of some of the pharmacologic actions of droperidol. *Toxicology and Applied Pharmacology* **6,** 37—47.

Yusa, T. (1973). Droperidol and pheochromocytoma. *Japanese Journal of Anaesthesia* **22,** 474—9.

10

Some clinical aspects

It is not proposed to discuss in detail the clinical use of intravenous anaesthetics but rather to present the pattern of their current use and contraindications, and to highlight their application in three fields where at one time it was widely held that they should not be used.

Intravenous anaesthesia became widely used in the early 1950s and has maintained its popularity as a means of inducing anaesthesia. As is pointed out in Chapter 11, it was originally regarded as a form of major general anaesthesia, rather than merely as a means of inducing sleep. Although there are no data on the actual use of individual agents, it is reasonable to assume that at least 95 per cent of adults who receive general anaesthesia today have an intravenous induction.

In a survey of 10000 patients scheduled for operation, Fee and his colleagues (1978) found that 6672 had had a previous anaesthetic. One-third of these stated that they had had an intravenous induction, but there were no data as to the nature of the drugs given. The agent was known in 2780 instances; the reported use was:

Barbiturate	80.4%
Althesin	18.1%
Ketamine	2.8%
Other intravenous	7.8%

On totalling, this exceeds 100 per cent but many patients had second anaesthetics and therefore had more than one induction agent. These figures would suggest that at the time (late 1976/early 1977) and place of survey, virtually all general anaesthetics included an intravenous induction. Too much attention should not be paid to the relative use of different agents, as this has obviously changed since the reports of hypersensitivity to Althesin. The 'other' intravenous agents used — in order of frequency — included droperidol - fentanyl, diazepam and propanidid. If prior use of an intravenous agent predisposes to hypersensitivity, then the widespread use of intravenous anaesthesia will create a major problem.

Are there any specific contraindications to intravenous anaesthetics in general or to individual drugs in particular? General contraindications do not change; for example, in a situation where control of the airway is impossible or where ventilation is maintained by the use of the accessory muscles, it is dangerous to rashly administer intravenous anaesthetics. Establishing a proper airway of course changes the whole pattern of events. Despite views to the contrary (Ward, 1965), a history of acute intermittent porphyria should still be an absolute contraindication to the use of thiopentone. Only a few sufferers will develop an acute attack but these carry about a 10 per cent mortality and the use of any barbiturate or Althesin is unjustified in these patients. One must now include a history of sensitivity to an intravenous drug as an absolute contraindication to its subsequent use.

Contraindications to the use of ketamine have been discussed in Chapter 5. It is not possible to be dogmatic about contraindications to Althesin: the author would avoid it in atopic patients, in those with a history of drug allergy and, if possible, when it had been administered previously.

There remain several clinical fields where extra caution and expertise in administration are indicated and where there is not a universal agreement as to the place of intravenous anaesthesia. These include paediatrics, obstetrics and cardiac surgery. Some anaesthetists would avoid using it completely, while others use it routinely. There follow three contributions in which colleagues who specialize in these branches express their personal views. These are not extensive reviews of world literature on the topics, but rather opinions based on practical experience. In the case of cardiac surgery, the place of intravenous morphine is reviewed and compared with conventional techniques.

Paediatrics S. R. Keilty

Children, especially those aged between 1 and 5 years, often experience great fear when forced to leave the security and comfort of their home to enter hospital. The induction of anaesthesia, especially if it is painful or traumatic, can produce psychological changes resulting in enuresis, temper tantrums and other behavioural problems. It is therefore surprising that the intravenous induction of anaesthesia has never achieved the same degree of popularity in paediatric practice as with adults. Except in large paediatric centres, anaesthesia — especially for the younger age groups — has usually been induced with inhalational agents. This lack of enthusiasm for intravenous anaesthesia has been due to the difficulties associated with venepuncture in small children and the dislike of needles often expressed by many older children who have experienced intramuscular injections. However, the skilful induction of anaesthesia by the intravenous route can be of great advantage to the child. A rapid, smooth induction is assured and the child is spared the relatively slow onset of anaesthesia which occurs even with modern inhalational agents.

Preoperative preparation and medication

An assessment of the physical and emotional state of the child should be made preoperatively and the presence of veins suitable for venepuncture should be noted. The emotional state of the child should be assessed and particular attention paid to those children having repeated procedures.

Children under 5 years suffer greatly from lack of security due to separation from their parents, while older children fear the pain and suffering from the operation they are about to undergo. Simple honest explanations as to the nature of the procedure and how they will be put to sleep do much to reassure the older child. However, calming the upset preschool child is much more difficult. The presence of a parent during the administration of premedicant drugs and, if possible, during the induction of anaesthesia can help to alleviate the emotional disturbances of this age group.

The stomach should be empty prior to the induction of anaesthesia but prolonged fasting should be avoided. Hypoglycaemia can occur, especially in children under 5 years. Clear fluids with glucose added should be allowed up to 4 hours before surgery in infants under 6 months and up to 6 hours in children between 6 months and 5 years.

Preanaesthetic medication

There is great variation in attitudes to preanaesthetic medication of children. Some anaesthetists prefer the child to be asleep on arrival in the operating room while others use little medication and rely on establishing rapport and creating an environment without fear. The preoperative visit should enable the anaesthetist to decide which particular approach to adopt.

It is widely accepted that infants under 1 year do not need preoperative sedation. Older infants and children are usually given some form of medication. Many drugs have been used for preanaesthetic medication and their number testify to their relative ineffectiveness. Morphine is perhaps the most popular drug being given intramuscularly in a dose of 0.2 $mg \cdot kg^{-1}$. It provides a reliable sedative effect and its analgesic action is of value postoperatively. A wide variety of sedatives has been advocated, either in combination with morphine or as the sole agent. Pentobarbitone given orally, rectally or intramuscularly* has been widely used in doses from 3 to 5 $mg \cdot kg^{-1}$ and trimeprazine tartrate, diazepam and triclofos have also been employed.

In the agitated preschool child the rectal administration of thiopentone or methohexitone can induce sleep prior to transfer to the operating room. However, the presence of an anaesthetist is necessary both to administer the drug and to supervise transfer of the child. Thiopentone can be given as either a 2.5 or 5 per cent solution in a dose of 30 $mg \cdot kg^{-1}$. Sleep will occur within 5—10 minutes. It has, until recently, been available as an emulsion in multidose calibrated syringes. Thiopentone suppositories are preferred by some but have to be given 45 minutes preoperatively.

Methohexitone in a 10 per cent solution has been given rectally in a dose of 20 $mg \cdot kg^{-1}$. The onset of sleep is rapid, occurring within 5 minutes, and postoperative recovery is not as prolonged as after thiopentone. It can also be given intramuscularly in doses of 6—7 $mg \cdot kg^{-1}$ with an onset time similar to that following rectal administration (Miller and Stoelting, 1963).

Most anaesthetists agree that the administration of an anti-cholinergic

*Preparation for parenteral administration is not available in the UK.

agent is advisable in children to provide a vagolytic effect and to prevent the bradycardia which can occur in response to painful surgical stimuli or after the administration of agents such as suxamethonium or halothane. Hyoscine has a better anti-sialogogue effect and greater sedative action than atropine but the abolition of vagal reflexes is more reliable with atropine, which is the author's drug of choice. Oral atropine has an unpredictable vagolytic effect and either the intramuscular or the intravenous route is preferred in a dose of 0.02 $mg \cdot kg^{-1}$ with a maximum dose of 0.6 mg.

Intravenous induction

Induction by the intravenous route ensures a smooth, rapid loss of consciousness without the struggling and crying which can arise with inhalational agents. It can be a relatively painless procedure if fine, 27 gauge needles are used. However, it does require dexterity on behalf of the anaesthetist and skilled assistance from the nursing staff.

Suitable veins can be found on the dorsum of the hand or foot, the volar aspect of the wrist, the antecubital fossa or on the scalp. However, care should be exercised when injecting irritant drugs into scalp veins as accidental intra-arterial injection can occur. When attempting venepuncture, the child should be gently but firmly held by an assistant who also compresses the arm. In small infants it is relatively easy to stop the arterial inflow by pressure, and blanching of the hand will occur. This should be avoided as venepuncture is made more difficult. The anaesthetist should firmly grip the arm or hand and stretch the skin over the venepuncture site. The older child is told that he is to have a 'little scratch' and at the moment of venepuncture has his attention distracted by the nurse, or he is asked to give a cough or a grunt.

Intravenous agents

Thiopentone

Thiopentone (2.5 per cent solution) is still the most popular agent for induction of anaesthesia in children, and is given in a dose of 3—5 $mg \cdot kg^{-1}$.

Methohexitone

Methohexitone (1 per cent solution) has been widely used for outpatient anaesthesia. It is given by slow injection in a dose of 1—1.5 $mg \cdot kg^{-1}$. However, children frequently complain of pain along the course of the vein during the injection. There is also a high incidence of muscle twitching and tremor and respiratory upset such as hiccough and coughing with this agent, especially when there is minimal preanaesthetic medication.

Propanidid

This agent is not recommended for small children as a large-bore needle is necessary for its administration. There is also a high incidence of post-operative nausea and vomiting, especially when followed by inhalational agents.

Althesin

This is administered in a dose of 50—75 $\mu l \cdot kg^{-1}$. The volume of solution required for children is small and this, coupled with absence of pain on injection and its non-irritant properties if injected extravascularly, would appear to offer advantages when used in paediatric practice. Some anaesthetists recommend diluting the drug to facilitate injection, but the author finds it simpler to use a small volume and a small syringe. Dilution reduces stability and such solutions should be used without delay. There have been reports of hypersensitivity reactions involving Althesin in children. One of these, in which the author was involved, was in an 8-year-old boy with a family history of asthma. His fourth anaesthetic, which was his second administration of Althesin, was followed by bronchoconstriction and hypotension. Children certainly are not immune from this frightening complication (Dundee *et al.*, 1974).

Ketamine

This has had widespread use in paediatric practice. It can be given intravenously or intramuscularly, producing analgesia without cardiovascular or respiratory depression and the airway is well maintained on most occasions.

Intravenous administration of 2 $mg \cdot kg^{-1}$ ketamine (1 per cent solution) will produce unconsciousness within 30 seconds. Vertical or horizontal nystagmus may be noted initially and when the eyes become central the patient is ready for surgery. This dose will last about 5—10 minutes. Muscle tone is enhanced and the airway is usually well maintained. There is little respiratory depressant effect and bronchodilation has been noted which may be of assistance when anaesthetizing children with asthma. Salivation can cause a problem and, unless an anti-sialogogue has been administered preoperatively, laryngeal spasm is likely to occur. The laryngeal reflexes are depressed and pulmonary aspiration has been reported. Instrumentation of the upper airway should be avoided because laryngeal spasm is likely to occur under ketamine anaesthesia. The intracranial pressure is greatly increased and ketamine is contraindicated when it is raised.

In early infancy (3—6 months) the effects of ketamine are very unpredictable. Large doses may be needed to produce satisfactory operating conditions and it is often associated with periods of apnoea and laryngospasm.

The psychomimetic side effects of ketamine, so commonly seen in adults, appear to be a less frequent occurrence in children.

Ketamine is a valuable drug in paediatric practice. It is especially useful for burn dressing and surgery, minor therapeutic procedures such as bone marrow aspirations, and radiological investigations. In most circumstances it is the drug of choice for repeat anaesthetics and the author has used it 25 times in one child. It can also be given intramuscularly (see Fig. 5.1) but care should be exercised that the injection is not too superficial.

Obstetrics J. Moore

Thirty years ago inhalation anaesthesia was the accepted method for pain relief in obstetrics. Balanced anaesthesia, involving narcosis, analgesia and muscle relaxation, despite its many advantages, was not employed because of lack of knowledge of the fetal effects of the drugs used. The finding that clinical doses of depolarizing or non-depolarizing relaxants did not cross the placenta in amounts sufficient to cause significant muscle weakness in the infant added a new impetus to the introduction of modern methods of anaesthesia to obstetrics. Present-day techniques rely on a light hypnotic—analgesic state in a totally paralysed patient and require judicious application if an unacceptable incidence of maternal awareness is to be avoided.

Awareness varies in severity from accurate intraoperative recall to non-specific dreaming. The choice and dosage of the intravenous induction agent will affect its incidence, being lowest with the thiobarbiturates and most frequent with the rapidly metabolized propanidid. These drugs are usually given in 'sleep' dosage, e.g. thiopentone sodium 4 $mg \cdot kg^{-1}$, followed by a paralysing dose of suxamethonium and rapid tracheal intubation. However, if this proves difficult and further inflation with oxygen is necessary, the risk of 'awake' intubation is greatly increased. Maintenance of 'light' anaesthesia continues until delivery of the baby is completed, the contribution of the induction agent to anaesthetic 'sleep' decreasing as the induction—delivery interval is prolonged. Awareness is much more likely if unsupplemented oxygen—nitrous oxide mixtures are used, whereas the addition of low concentrations of trichloroethylene, halothane or methoxyflurane will greatly reduce the danger (Moir, 1970; Crawford, 1971; Crawford and Davies, 1975). This complication is also more frequent in the unpremedicated patient for elective surgery and is rare in the parturient who has received sedative—analgesic treatment. The role of the benzodiazepines in minimizing the risk of recall is discussed in Chapter 7.

Active vomiting following intravenous anaesthetics is much less common than with inhalation agents. However, regurgitation of gastric contents can occur especially when suxamethonium is given as this increases intragastric pressure. The induction agents — with the possible exception of ketamine — depress the protective laryngeal reflex (Carson *et al.*, 1973) and this effect is enhanced by sedative—analgesic premedication. The danger to the obstetric patient of soiling the lung with highly acid gastric contents is well known, hence most authorities now recommend tracheal intubation when intravenous anaesthesia is used.

The supine hypotensive syndrome (Scott, 1968) is a well recognized problem in late pregnancy. All intravenous induction agents, except ketamine, depress the cardiovascular system and will accentuate existing hypotension or, by impairing compensatory mechanisms, unmask the syndrome. Lateral tilting will remove the pressure effect of the pregnant uterus on the inferior vena cava, restoring venous return, cardiac output, blood pressure and placental perfusion. Ketamine, because of its cardiostimulatory effects, may be used to induce anaesthesia in patients with pre-existing supine hypotension (Bunodière *et al.*, 1977).

None of the currently available intravenous agents depresses uterine function or increases the incidence of placental retention or third stage blood loss. Ketamine may increase uterine tone and make intrauterine manipulation more difficult (Dick *et al.*, 1973).

All these drugs are readily transferred through the placenta to the infant. Large doses administered to the mother will increase the incidence of sleepy depressed infants, which are marked if maternal hypotension and respiratory depression are untreated. Kosaka, Takahashi and Mark (1969) reported that, following an induction dose of 4 $mg{\cdot}kg^{-1}$ of thiopentone, 90 per cent of infants had Apgar scores of 7–10 as compared with 60 per cent when the dose of the intravenous agent was doubled. These workers demonstrated measurable quantities of drug in the infant 45 seconds after maternal administration and peak values at 90–180 seconds depending on dose and rate of administration. The drug concentrations noted in the umbilical vein are not necessarily the concentration arriving at the fetal brain. Indeed, a large part of the umbilical venous blood goes through the liver which extracts substantial amounts of thiobarbiturate entering the fetus (Finster *et al.*, 1967). The maternal blood concentration falls rapidly after a single dose of intravenous anaesthetic so that continued drug transfer is greatly reduced.

Intravenous anaesthetics with shorter duration of action and less cumulative effect have been evaluated in obstetrics. Methohexitone (Holdcroft *et al.*, 1974), propanidid (Downing, Coleman and Meer, 1972), Althesin (Downing *et al.*, 1974; Holdcroft *et al.*, 1975) and ketamine (Marx, 1977) have all been used but marked advantages to the infant have not been demonstrated. More detailed and prolonged assessment of the neonate as suggested by Dubowitz (1975) may show a particular drug to be significantly better than the others.

Intravenous induction agents, because of their sedative and anti-convulsant actions, are sometimes used in the management of eclamptic states. The aim is to induce a light plane of narcosis where the patient is just rousable and supports her own airway. Rapid administration will produce deep sedation, hypotension and respiratory depression. Chlormethiazole and diazepam are the most commonly used drugs. Duffus *et al.* (1969) reported good maternal effects from chlormethiazole without associated severe infant depression. Diazepam, whilst producing satisfactory sedative effects in the mother, can, if given in excessive dosage, cause infant hypotoxicity and exacerbation of neonatal jaundice (Moir, 1976).

The intravenous induction agents have contributed greatly to patient acceptability of anaesthesia in obstetrics. Their safe use demands expert anaesthetic care so that mother and infant are spared the harmful effects of mismanagement or overdosage.

Cardiac surgery I. W. Carson

In the last decade common practice was to prefer a light-plane of general anaesthesia with halothane or methoxyflurane, possibly supplemented with small doses of intravenous analgesics in adults and children undergoing cardiac surgery. Induction of anaesthesia in adults was most frequently instituted by the intravenous route, using thiopentone or methohexitone. In children with congenital heart disease inhalation induction was usually preferred, although intravenous or intramuscular ketamine temporarily achieved a degree of popularity.

However, there has been a recent trend — especially in North America and Europe — to replace fluorinated inhalation anaesthetics with intravenous techniques employing morphine and morphine-like drugs.

Clinical observations of the minimal haemodynamic alterations produced by morphine given postoperatively or as a preoperative medication led Lowenstein and his colleagues (1969) in Boston to use large doses of morphine (0.5—3.0 $mg{\cdot}kg^{-1}$) as the sole anaesthetic or in combination with inhalation anaesthetic agents in patients undergoing open-heart surgery. Studies revealed that 1 $mg{\cdot}kg^{-1}$ morphine administered intravenously did not affect cardiac output, systemic vascular resistance, blood pressure, central venous pressure or pulse rate in healthy man, but uniformly decreased systemic vascular resistance and increased cardiac output in patients with impaired myocardial function.

As this high-dose morphine technique of 'anaesthesia' achieved moderate popularity, it became apparent that, whereas morphine guaranteed profound analgesia, there was no reliable indication that the patient would be 'asleep' and remain amnesic (Lowenstein, 1971). This became particularly apparent in patients with unimpaired left ventricular performance. The addition of nitrous oxide to morphine anaesthesia, to provide amnesia, has been demonstrated to cause cardiovascular depression (Wong *et al.*, 1973). Furthermore, Stoelting and his colleagues (1974) demonstrated that the addition of low concentrations of halothane to morphine (1 $mg{\cdot}kg^{-1}$) anaesthesia produced progressive decreases in mean arterial pressure, heart rate, stroke volume and cardiac index.

Hypotension may occur during induction of anaesthesia with high dose of morphine, particularly if the rate of administration is too rapid. This can be readily corrected by transfusion of crystalloid solutions and, if necessary, elevation of the patient's legs. As a result of the increase in total vascular capacitance it has been demonstrated that patients anaesthetized with high-dose morphine may require significantly more blood during bypass than patients anaesthetized with halothane—nitrous oxide (Stanley *et al.*, 1974).

The maintenance of cardiac output in the presence of a decreased peripheral vascular resistance following high-dose morphine anaesthesia has been attributed to the liberation of endogenous noradrenaline and adrenaline in man (Hasbrouck, 1970). Hypertension during morphine anaesthesia may occur in some patients, particularly those for aorto-coronary bypass surgery, following skin incision or sternotomy. The use of sodium nitroprusside, or other such agent to decrease the 'afterload' on the myocardium, will control the hypertension and prevent an increase in myocardial oxygen consumption.

The current practice in the author's unit is to administer morphine in a dose of 2 mg·kg^{-1} and at a rate not greater than 10 mg·min^{-1} by a volumetric infusion pump. In addition, diazepam (0.5 mg·kg^{-1}) is given to ensure sleep and absence of recall. Following curarization and endotracheal intubation, the patient is ventilated with oxygen-enriched air. No additional anaesthesia has been found necessary to cover the cardiopulmonary bypass period.

This technique, apart from its beneficial effects on the circulatory system, enables a smooth transition to elective postoperative ventilator support. The patients are comfortable, tolerating the endotracheal tube well, and remain pain-free for long periods postoperatively, requiring less frequent and lower doses of sedative drugs.

There is a preference in other centres for the neuroleptic combination of droperidol and fentanyl, drugs which cause minimal myocardial depression combined with an alpha-adrenergic blocking property.

Anaesthesia can be induced with these drugs alone, to a total dose of approximately 100 μg·kg^{-1} droperidol and 10 μg·kg^{-1} fentanyl using increments of 2.5—5.0 mg droperidol and 0.125—0.25 mg fentanyl. Smaller increments of these drugs may be employed following induction with an intravenous barbiturate. Short-acting intravenous inductions agents have little or no benefit for patients undergoing open-heart surgery.

References

Bunodière, M., Green, M., Bunodière, N., Ravaud, Y., Guilmet, C. and Deligné, P. (1977). Ketamine hydrochloride and obstetric anesthesia. In: *Clinical use of Ketamine in Obstetrical and Gynecological Indications,* Selected Proceedings of the Sixth World Congress of Anaesthesiology, Mexico City, April 24—30 1976, pp. 27—33. Excerpta Medica, Amsterdam.

Carson, I. W., Moore, J., Balmer, J. P., Dundee, J. W. and McNabb, T. G. (1973). Laryngeal competence with ketamine. *Anesthesiology* **38,** 128—33.

Crawford, J. S. (1971). Awareness during operative obstetrics under general anaesthesia. *British Journal of Anaesthesia* **43,** 179—82.

Crawford, J. S. and Davies, P. (1975). A return to trichloroethylene for obstetric anaesthesia. *British Journal of Anaesthesia* **47,** 482—90.

Dick, W., Borst, R., Fodor, H., Haug, H., Milewki, H., Schumann, R. and Traub, E. (1973). Ketamine in obstetrical anesthesia: clinical and experimental results. *Journal of Perinatal Medicine* **1,** 252—62.

Downing, J. W., Coleman, A. J. and Meer, F. M. (1972). An intravenous method of anaesthesia for Caesarean section. Part 1: Propanidid. *British Journal of Anaesthesia* **44,** 1069—76.

Downing, J. W., Mahomedy, M. C., Coleman, A. J., Mahomedy, Y. H. and Jeal, D. E. (1974). Anaesthetic induction for Caesarean section: Althesin versus thiopentone. *Anaesthesia* **29,** 689—95.

Dubowitz, V. (1975). Neurological fragility in the newborn: influenced by medication in labour. *British Journal of Anaesthesia* **47,** 1005—10.

Duffus, G. M., Tunstall, M. E., Condie, R. G. and McGillivray, I. (1969). Chlormethiazole in the prevention of eclampsia and the reduction of perinatal mortality. *Journal of Obstetrics and Gynaecology of the British Commonwealth* **76,** 645—51.

Dundee, J. W., Assem, E. S. K., Gaston, J. H., Keilty, S. R., Sutton, J. A., Clarke, R. S. J. and Grainger, D. (1974). Sensitivity to intravenous anaesthetics: report of three cases. *British Medical Journal* **1,** 63—5.

Fee, J. P. H., McDonald, J. R., Dundee, J. W. and Clarke, R. S. J. (1978). Frequency of previous anaesthesia in an anaesthetic population. *British Journal of Anaesthesia* **50,** 917—20.

Finster, M., Morishima, A., Mark, L. C. and Dayton, P. G. (1967). Distribution of thiopental in fetal tissues. *Obstetrics and Gynecology* **29,** 440.

Hasbrouck, J. D. (1970). Morphine anesthesia for open heart surgery. *Annals of Thoracic Surgery* **10,** 364—9.

Holdcroft, A., Morgan, M., Gordon, H., Whitwam, J. G. and White, Y. (1975). Althesin as an induction agent for Caesarean section. *British Journal of Anaesthesia* **47,** 1213—17.

Holdcroft, A., Robinson, M. J., Gordon, H. and Whitwam, J. G. (1974). Comparison of effect of two induction doses of methohexitone on infants delivered by elective Caesarean section. *British Medical Journal* **2,** 472—5.

Kosaka, Y., Takahashi, T. and Mark, L. C. (1969). Intravenous thiobarbiturate anesthesia for caesarean section. *Anesthesiology* **31,** 489—506.

Lowenstein, E. (1971). Morphine anesthesia — a perspective. *Anesthesiology* **35,** 563—5.

Lowenstein, E., Hallowell, P., Levine, F. H., Daggett, W. M., Austen, W. G. and Laver, M. B. (1969). Cardiovascular response to large doses of intravenous morphine in man. *New England Journal of Medicine* **281,** 1389—93.

Marx, G. F. (1977). Ketamine in obstetrics and gynecology — 1976. In: *Clinical use of Ketamine in Obstetrical and Gynecological Indications,* Selected Proceedings of the Sixth World Congress of Anaesthesiology, Mexico City, April 24—30 1976, pp. 1—14. Excerpta Medica, Amsterdam.

Miller, J. R. and Stoelting, V. K. (1963). A preliminary communication of the sleep-producing effect of intramuscular methohexitone sodium in the paediatric patient. *British Journal of Anaesthesia* **35,** 48—50.

Moir, D. D. (1970). Anaesthesia for caesarean section. *British Journal of Anaesthesia* **42,** 136—42.

Moir, D. D. (1976). *Obstetric Anaesthesia and Analgesia,* 1st edn., p. 49. Bailliere Tindall, London.

Scott, D. B. (1968). Inferior vena caval occlusion in late pregnancy and its importance in anaesthesia. *British Journal of Anaesthesia* **40,** 120—8.

Stanley, T. H., Gray, N. H., Isern-Amaral, J. H. and Patton, C. (1974). Comparison of blood requirements during morphine and halothane anesthesia for open-heart surgery. *Anesthesiology* **41,** 34—8.

Stoelting, R. K., Creasser, C. W., Gibbs, P. S. and Peterson, C. (1974). Circulatory effects of halothane added to morphine anesthesia in patients with coronary artery disease. *Anesthesia and Analgesia . . . Current Researches* **53**, 449—55.

Ward, R. J. (1965). Porphyria and its relation to anesthesia. *Anesthesiology* **26**, 212—15.

Wong, K. C., Martin, W. E., Hornbein, T. F., Freund, F. G. and Everett, J. (1973). The cardiovascular effects of morphine sulphate with oxygen and with nitrous oxide in man. *Anesthesiology* **38**, 542—9.

11

Total intravenous anaesthesia

When hexobarbitone and thiopentone were introduced into anaesthetic practice it was anticipated that they would be used as sole agents for total anaesthesia. This was the then currently accepted use of ether and chloroform. The first recorded clinical administration of thiopentone, on 6 March 1935, was of 600 mg (of 10 per cent) given as sole agent for the insertion of radium into the tongue. One can look back at this anaesthetic and appreciate that it could have ended disastrously with inhalation of blood, laryngospasm or respiratory obstruction, and possibly with the abandonment — at least for a time — of this agent. Fortunately, all went well and a new era in anaesthesia had begun. With the introduction of the intravenous barbiturate one had a simple, rapid and compact method of producing general anaesthesia. It would seem to offer much in circumstances where portability was an advantage.

However, as the popularity of thiopentone increased and its use extended, the dangers of total intravenous anaesthesia began to be appreciated. Following the Japanese air raid on Pearl Harbour on 9 December 1941, hexobarbitone and thiopentone were given as sole agents to war casualties with such disastrous results as to be called 'an ideal form of euthanasia' (Halford, 1943). Judged by present-day standards it will be appreciated that the lack of trained personnel and an inadequate knowledge of the actions of the drugs involved were the main factors involved in this tragedy. In the same issue of *Anesthesiology* which carried the critique on intravenous anaesthesia in war casualties, there was a report of its safe use in one seriously shocked patient with a gunshot wound. Adams and Gray (1943) reported that the use of small doses of very dilute solutions given slowly made thiopentone safer in shocked patients but the concept of 'total intravenous anaesthesia' still persisted. Thiopentone was looked on as a substitute for ether, capable of doing all that the inhalation agent did. The toxicity of large doses, given either to produce relaxation and deep anaesthesia or over an extended period for prolonged narcosis, was not fully appreciated.

An example of the toxicity of large doses of barbiturates was the use of a thiopentone infusion as an anti-convulsant sedative in eclampsia (O'Donel Browne, 1950). In this it was successful but, although the frequency of convulsions was markedly reduced, the mortality was not lowered as cardiovascular depression from large doses of thiopentone became the main cause of death. Another similar use was to control the convulsions of tetanus (Grant and McNeilly, 1953); although there are no reported deaths from its use in this field, it did not gain widespread acceptance.

It is difficult to trace the evolution of the use of the 'induction dose' of barbiturates as part of a balanced anaesthetic technique; the advocacy of the concomitant use of nitrous oxide—oxygen with intermittent thiopentone by Organe and Broad in 1938 was a major step in the right direction. The reduction of the dose of barbiturate required for a prolonged anaesthesia made the balanced technique more acceptable for a wide variety of patients of varying degrees of fitness.

The introduction of myoneural blocking drugs and halothane paved the way for the rational use of an intravenous induction agent as we know it today. It is often forgotten that a greater knowledge of the basic pharmacology of each of these drugs has also played a part in developing this rational approach. Appreciation of the concept of dose-related (or tissue-concentration-related) toxicity, of 'acute tolerance' (with consequent reduction in dosage), of the lack of analgesic action of the barbiturates and an understanding of their pharmacokinetics has played a major role in safer use of intravenous anaesthetics.

Much of the knowledge of intravenous anaesthetics which is now taken for granted has been obtained at the cost of a high morbidity, and even mortality, resulting from early misuse. Thiopentone — perhaps one of the most dangerous drugs available in modern medicine — has been 'tamed' by an appreciation of its limitations and toxicity and by delineating principles for its safe use. One hopes that the lessons learnt in this process will not be forgotten in the current upsurge of interest in total intravenous anaesthesia.

The development of shorter-acting, less cumulative and, it is hoped, less toxic intravenous anaesthetics, coming at a time when theatre pollution by gases and vapours is becoming a topic of some concern, has been the prelude to renewed interest in total intravenous anaesthesia. It is the only available method for the complete elimination of pollution. Basically, it consists of the continuous infusion of a sufficient dose of an intravenous anaesthetic to produce and maintain the desired degree of sedation or anaesthesia. It may be preceded by a bolus dose, with additional small increments as required. The patient may be breathing oxygen, air or oxygen-enriched air and curarized in appropriate circumstances. A further addition is the concomitant use of narcotic analgesics.

Ketamine, Althesin and etomidate would appear to be drugs most suitable for this technique. By virtue of its prolonged action, minute to minute control of the 'depth' of narcosis is most difficult with ketamine but it has a good analgesic action which commends it for this use (Chapter 5). Easy control of the degree of cerebral depression and a very rapid return of consciousness have been features of the continuous use of Althesin which seems an ideal drug for this purpose (Savege *et al.*, 1975). The high incidence of induction side effects which detract from the usefulness of etomidate as a routine intravenous anaesthetic (Chapter 6) may not be a problem with continuous administration when it is combined with narcotic analgesia and/or myoneural blocking drugs.

Attractive as is the concept of total intravenous anaesthesia, let us not forget the lessons which were learnt from the early use of the barbiturates as sole anaesthetic agent. While ketamine, Althesin and etomidate may not have the same cardiovascular depressant action as thiopentone, their effects in high doses should be investigated. Likewise, one must not assume that large doses of drugs which are broken down by the liver would not have a hepatotoxic action. It has been convincingly demonstrated that in large doses both thiopentone and propanidid cause enzyme changes which are generally regarded as being indicative of liver dysfunction. Similar changes frequently occur when ketamine is infused for intermediate types of operation of 20—40 minutes' duration, but are not found with conventional techniques. However, enzyme changes have not been found when similar large doses (up to 6 $mg \cdot kg^{-1}$) are given as sole agent for minor gynaecological operations. Liver dysfunction has not been found after very large doses or continuous infusion of etomidate (Chapter 6). The situation is less clear with Althesin for, although there has been evidence of enzyme changes following continuous infusions for long-term sedation, these occurred in patients who were receiving other drugs and in whom there were other possible explanations for the findings.

One has to examine the evidence of toxicity with clinical perspective. Despite the biochemical findings of liver dysfunction with ketamine, there has been no reported case of jaundice, nor as yet are we certain as to the exact significance of the enzyme changes. However, one should be cautious with large doses of drugs in patients undergoing intermediate types of operation; this warning should also apply to Althesin and to etomidate. This highlights one of the problems in the evaluation of continuous intravenous anaesthesia because doses which have no apparent toxicity when given for minor operations may prove unsafe when the peritoneum is opened or the patient is subjected to other stresses. We need to consider this possibility when evaluating the toxicity of every proposed technique.

The effect of large amounts of the solvents used in some commercial preparations of intravenous anaesthetics must also be considered. This was not a problem with the barbiturates, nor does it apply to ketamine. We must, however, be certain that, in the doses used for total intravenous anaesthesia, the solubilizing agent used in Althesin and the inorganic solvent which will eventually be used with etomidate are both free from tissue toxicity and do not have a haemolytic action. The intravascular haemolysis which resulted from the solvent used when large intravenous doses of mephenesin were employed as a muscle relaxant must not be forgotten (Mallinson, 1948).

Continuous intravenous sedation

Chlormethiazole, a vitamin B derivative which was once investigated as an intravenous anaesthetic under the designation of SCTZ, can be given continuously in a commercially available 0.8 per cent solution (Heminevrin). Rapid infusion can induce and maintain anaesthesia but its clinical application is as a sedative or anti-convulsant, particularly in eclampsia.

Just as the apparent simplicity of administration led to the use of thiopentone by those who were both unaware of and unable to deal with its dangerous side effects, so there is still a possibility that the infusion of these potent drugs in smaller doses in order to produce sedation could be given by staff not fully conversant with their toxicity. It would seem an attractive hypothesis to have virtual fingertip control of sedation of patients by this means. However, in inexpert hands, the widespread use of continuous intravenous sedation would inevitably lead to disasters. Continuous intravenous sedation is nothing less than continuous intravenous anaesthesia, with all its hazards (Dundee, 1978).

References

Adams, R. C. and Gray, H. K. (1943). Intravenous anesthesia with pentothal sodium in the case of gunshot wound associated with accompanying severe traumatic shock and loss of blood: report of a case. *Anesthesiology* **4,** 70—3.

Dundee, J. W. (1978). Total intravenous anaesthesia. *British Journal of Anaesthesia* **50,** 89—90.

Grant, A. P. and McNeilly, J. W. (1953). Treatment of tetanus with intravenous thiopentone and pethidine. *Irish Journal of Medical Science,* 6th Series, 212—17.

Halford, F. J. (1943). A critique of intravenous anesthesia in war surgery. *Anesthesiology* **4,** 67—9.

Mallinson, F. B. (1948). Present position of Myanesin in anaesthesia: clinical aspects. *Proceedings of the Royal Society of Medicine* **41,** 593—606.

O'Donel Browne (1950). The treatment of eclampsia. *Journal of Obstetrics and Gynaecology of the British Empire* **57,** 573—82.

Organe, G. S. W. and Broad, R. J. B. (1938). Pentothal with nitrous oxide and oxygen. *Lancet* **ii,** 1170—2.

Savege, T. M., Ramsay, M. A. E., Curran, J. P. J., Cotter, J., Walling, P. T. and Simpson, B. R. (1975). Intravenous anaesthesia by infusion: a technique using alphaxalone/alphadolone (Althesin). *Anaesthesia* **30,** 757—64.

12

The ideal intravenous anaesthetic(s)

Much has been written on this subject: in fact, the introduction of each new intravenous anaesthetic seems to have sparked off a spate of publications on the properties of the ideal agent. In the final chapter of a book on current topics in the field of intravenous anaesthesia it would seem appropriate to consider once again the desirable properties of an ideal agent. There can be no universal agreement on this subject because personal preferences and experience will influence one's priorities. Some of the views expressed here are naturally the personal preferences of the author. It is possible that we should be looking for more than one agent to satisfy all our needs.

Physical properties

The greatest agreement relates to the physical properties the ideal agent (Table 12.1). Organic solvents and lipophilic agents produce viscid solutions which have a tendency to froth and are messy to handle. In addition, the non-anaesthetic component is not always free from side effects, of which hypersensitivity and intravascular haemolysis are the most important. Prolonged stability of solutions is probably less important than has been suggested. For many years we have become used to preparing solutions of barbiturates prior to induction — this has not caused any insurmountable problems. Few would object to a new agent which is prepared in ampoules in powder form but all would almost certainly prefer a solution which is more stable than thiopentone. Rather than a longer 'shelf' life, we would like a longer 'bench' life. This means a solution which is less alkaline than the barbiturates and which would not interact with atmospheric

Table 12.1 Some properties of an ideal intravenous anaesthetic

1. Water soluble
2. Stable in solution
3. Long shelf life
4. No pain on intravenous injection
5. Non-irritant on subcutaneous injection
6. Painful on arterial injection
7. No sequelae from arterial injection of small amounts
8. Low incidence of venous thrombosis
9. Small volume of isotonic solution required for induction

Table 12.2 Physical and other properties of six available drugs compared with those of the ideal intravenous anaesthetic

Properties	Thiopentone	Methohexitone	Propanidid	Althesin	Ketamine	Etomidate
Water soluble	+	+	−	−	+	+
Stable in solution	−	−		+	+	
Long shelf life	−	−		+	+	
No pain on intravenous injection	+	−	+	+	+	−
Non-irritant on subcutaneous injection	−	±	+	+	+	
Painful on arterial injection	+	+		−		
No sequelae from intra-arterial injection	−	±	+	+		
Low incidence of thrombosis	+	+	−	+	+	−
Small volume	−	+ (2%)	±	+	+	−

carbon dioxide. One would hope that such a solution would be less irritant on extravenous injection. Ideally, an anaesthetic should be effective by both the intravenous and intramuscular routes; with such a drug a lower ratio of intramuscular to intravenous dose than the 3—4 : 1 of ketamine would be a safety factor in the event of very rapid absorption of the intramuscular injection. We have no knowledge as to why certain aqueous solutions such as methohexitone should cause pain along the course of the vein but obviously this is undesirable.

It is imperative that, in the rare event of intra-arterial injection, a small dose of the ideal intravenous anaesthetic should not cause spasm or thrombosis. The occurrence of pain on an arterial injection can be helpful as it permits early recognition of the accident and the injection can be stopped. It is unlikely that no sequelae will occur if large doses of drug which produce pain on arterial injection would cause some tissue damage.

Although painless thrombosis may do no harm, theoretically the risk of embolism is always present and often it is preceded by painful thrombophlebitis. One would therefore prefer an agent which produces a very low incidence of thrombosis. Clearly, no venous sequelae is an impossibility as the act of venepuncture and withdrawal of blood occasionally cause vascular damage and phlebitis.

There is much to be said for the use of a small syringe for injection. This makes easier the use of small needles and small veins. If an adult anaesthetic dose of isotonic solution could be less than 5 ml this would be very desirable, but it is not an essential prerequisite of an ideal intravenous anaesthetic. It does, however increase the risk of overdose from too rapid injection.

On the above criteria, the physical properties of methohexitone are the nearest to the ideal intravenous anaesthetic. Pain on injection is its only disadvantage (Table 12.2).

Onset

For easy control of dosage and to minimize the risk of overdosage, a drug which produces its action in one arm—brain circulation time is clearly desirable. This does carry the risk of a 'bolus' action on the cardiovascular and respiratory systems, and also sudden relaxation of sphincters and increased risk of aspiration of vomitus. Nevertheless, the advantages of rapid onset more than outweigh the disadvantages of a drug which is used primarily for induction. The pharmacokinetics of drug action are such that an agent with a quick onset of action will also leave the brain rapidly and recovery will be quicker than with slower-acting drugs.

There may be a place for a drug with a slower onset of action to be used as a basal anaesthetic. Its main uses would be for long operations and as a sedative in patients receiving artificial ventilation in an intensive therapy situation. The extremely slow onset of hydroxydione, a compound which probably had first to be converted to an active anaesthetic in the body, was unacceptable but the 30—90 seconds' delay with ketamine or diazepam is usually acceptable.

Recovery

It is desirable for recovery from the effect of the drug to result from both translocation to non-nervous tissue and rapid detoxication. Such a drug will be less cumulative than one which relies mainly on redistribution. Any metabolite(s) should not have a hypnotic action.

With such a compound, patients will awake with a very little unchanged drug in the body and there will be a lesser risk of 'reinduction' of anaesthesia following the administration of sedatives or analgesics in the postoperative period. Equally important, outpatients will not be at risk should they take alcohol in the early postoperative period.

Having had experience with propanidid, one is aware of the dangers of a too-short-acting drug. Time is required for the onset of action of gaseous and volatile agents following induction of anaesthesia by an intravenous agent. A recovery which is too rapid carries the risk of the patient recalling tracheal intubation. Even when used as a sole or principal agent for minor procedures, recovery can be too rapid. There is a risk of trying to prolong the duration of anaesthesia by giving larger doses of drug, and this can lead to a dangerous degree of cardiovascular or respiratory depression.

Analgesia

Apart from ketamine, none of the induction agents has a potent analgesic action. One feels that this would be desirable, but analgesia must not be 'bought' at the price of undesirable side effects. It has often been stated that analgesia, respiratory depression and vomiting are inseparable as far as a drug's activity is concerned but ketamine has demonstrated that this is not true. If analgesia cannot be produced by small doses of the induction agent, then an increase in sensitivity to somatic pain must be avoided; i.e. it must not possess an antanalgesic or hyperalgesic action.

An agent producing an analgesic action which persisted into the early postoperative period would be very useful for major operations.

Induction complications

Excitatory effects (tremor, spontaneous involuntary muscle movements and hypertonus) are undesirable effects of intravenous anaesthetics. Generally, the incidence and severity of these are related to dosage and the rate of injection. It is unlikely that any general anaesthetic will be free from some involuntary muscle movements but these must not reach an unacceptably high incidence or be of such severity as to make induction of anaesthesia difficult. A degree of hypertonus which interferes with positioning of the patient would be completely unacceptable in a new intravenous anaesthetic.

Coughing and hiccough are undesirable complications of any induction agent. Their incidence and severity are, to some extent, dose-related. Again, it is unlikely that any new anaesthetic will be free of such side effects, but a low incidence is desirable and it is important that they should not persist during the operation. Laryngeal spasm, at one time a dreaded complication of thiopentone, is no longer a problem; however, it is possible that a drug with marked vagotonic properties might cause disturbing salivation in the absence of an anti-sialogogue. This is probably an inevitable complication of anaesthesia but it would be advantageous to be able to avoid anti-sialogogue premedication, especially in small children.

Respiratory and cardiovascular effects

The mere fact that a patient loses consciousness and contact with his environment will itself produce some depression of respiration. Similarly, there is inevitably a small fall in arterial pressure and often in heart rate. To hope for a drug which produces no cardiovascular or respiratory depression is unrealistic. The ideal intravenous anaesthetic should have a favourable cardiovascular dose-response relationship with respect to its depressant effects. Some vasodilatation is desirable with the induction of anaesthesia and, although this will make hypovolaemic patients more susceptible to falls in the systolic blood pressure, this complication can readily be dealt with and overcome by suitable infusions or transfusions. Some degree of direct myocardial depression is likewise probably unavoidable with any anaesthetic, but this can be compensated for by liberation of catecholamine and its effect should be minimal with induction doses. The part played by direct myocardial depression in the production of hypotension is always more significant at larger dose levels and with repeated injections. An advantageous dose-response effect relative to the hypnotic effect is desirable. Propanidid is an example of a drug with an undesirable dose response curve; small doses cause about the same degree of hypotension as equivalent amounts of thiopentone, but doubling the dose produces much more depression with propanidid. In contrast, Althesin has a particularly good dose-response effect as far as cardiovascular depression is concerned. It is debatable whether there is any advantage in having a drug with the cardio-stimulatory action of ketamine; some release of catecholamines would minimize the direct depressant effects but a drug which consistently causes a rise of 20—40 mmHg in systolic pressure is clearly undesirable. Tachycardia is also an undesirable action in an ideal anaesthetic, yet despite this there has been an absence of reports incriminating the tachycardia which inevitably follows methohexitone and ketamine as a cause of cardiac failure. Clearly, a drug which produces tachycardia would be unsuitable in cardiac surgery and should be avoided in certain patients. Cardiovascular effects secondary to histamine release are also undesirable — the response frequently seen with intravenous pethidine is unacceptable in a new agent. The anaphylactoid response with profound hypotension is discussed later.

As a group, the intravenous anaesthetics do not produce gross disturbance of cardiac rhythm, apart from tachydysrhythmias with propanidid. The incidence of these with thiopentone or Althesin is clinically acceptable and these drugs approach the properties of the ideal agent in this respect. Although it may seem a remote possibility, an intravenous anaesthetic which sensitizes the myocardium to the effect of adrenaline would not be acceptable. This would not only limit the use of vasoconstrictors or vasopressors, but would also be likely to cause carbon-dioxide-induced dysrhythmias.

Although the initial respiratory stimulant action of propanidid has been used to advantage for blind nasal intubation, this is not an attribute which one would seek in a new agent. It would be preferable to have an agent which would not depress the normal response to carbon dioxide, provided that the depressant effects of the narcotic analgesics would not be synergistic.

In relation to the total picture of properties of an ideal intravenous anaesthetic, the author does not rate the absence of cardiovascular and/or respiratory depression high on the list of priorities. A compound with a marked direct depressant action should not pass the stage of animal screening. We have learnt to live with the depressant effects of thiopentone, methohexitone and Althesin; if a new compound were at least as good as the latter of these, and was otherwise acceptable, it certainly would not be unsuitable for consideration as an ideal intravenous anaesthetic.

Muscular relaxation

One might list the production of muscular relaxation as a desirable property but there are two clearly delineated viewpoints; this may point to the need for two ideal intravenous anaesthetics. One would not want a drug with a curare-like myoneural blocking action, neither would one like jaw relaxation of sufficient degree to permit tracheal intubation as this would increase the risk of respiratory obstruction.

The maintenance of jaw tone, with easy control of the airway, such as occurs with ketamine, is a desirable feature but it must not be achieved at the cost of marked generalized hypertonus. It is unlikely that such an agent would be suitable for minor procedures such as reduction of fractures but it would be useful for induction prior to an inhalational gaseous—volatile agent sequence. A mephenesin-like action, on intranuncial neurones in the spinal cord, would enable a drug to be used as sole agent for manipulations, examination under anaesthesia, and so on, without producing respiratory depression. It is worth noting that most (if not all) drugs with this type of action are insoluble in water, and if this is a prerequisite to a central muscular relaxing action then it should not be considered an essential for an ideal intravenous anaesthetic. Perhaps one ideal drug may produce muscular relaxation by a direct action of the anaesthetic on striated muscle.

Uterine muscle tone should not be affected by a normal induction dose of the ideal intravenous anaesthetic. However, the ability to produce transient relaxation of the uterus with large doses of drug would be of value in certain circumstances, but it would not be an essential property of an ideal agent. An action on smooth muscle is also non-essential; it is more important that stimulation of the muscle should not occur lest bronchospasm be produced.

Intravenous anaesthetics should not interact with neuromuscular blocking drugs nor should they be dependent on the cholinesterase group of enzymes for their inactivation. The propanidid—procaine—suxamethonium—plasma—cholinesterase interactions are best avoided in a new drug.

It is essential that an ideal intravenous anaesthetic should not increase serum potassium levels if it is to be used with suxamethonium. Since one would not wish to have an induction agent which is unsuitable for use prior to a depolarizing relaxant, there is no place for a new intravenous anaesthetic which liberates potassium from the muscles. Ideally, the agent should encourage the passage of K^+ into cells and thus make safer its combination with suxamethonium in burned patients and in those with a similar metabolic disturbance.

Other desiderata

The ideal intravenous anaesthetic must not induce malignant hyperpyrexia in susceptible patients; in fact, it should protect against its occurrence. Neither will it affect ALA synthetase and induce acute intermittent porphyria. The production of methaemoglobinaemia or sulphaemoglobinaemia is obviously an undesirable action of an ideal induction agent.

If a drug maintains a stable blood pressure by an increase in circulating catecholamines, then it is likely to cause a slight degree of hyperglycaemia. The emphasis must be on the extent of the rise in blood sugar as a marked hyperglycaemic action is not desirable.

An intravenous anaesthetic which increases cerebral blood flow and raises intracranial pressure is limited in its clinical uses. Ideally, we would prefer a drug which decreases cerebral metabolism to a greater degree than cerebral flow because this would give some degree of protection against hypoxia, particularly in hypotensive states.

Intraocular pressure should also be unaffected or even slightly lowered by the ideal intravenous anaesthetic. It must not affect the action of atropine or similar drugs on the eye.

Although it is not known whether a single short exposure to a drug can affect a fetus, the ideal intravenous anaesthetic should be free from teratogenicity. Animal experiments will have shown the effects of prolonged or repeated administration of the drug, and if there is any suspicion as to its toxic action on the developing fetus, the drug should not be used.

Hypersensitivity reactions

To state that an ideal intravenous anaesthetic should never produce an anaphylactoid attack is probably being quite unrealistic. The incidence and severity of hypersensitivity reactions must be very low, even in atopic patients and those who show a sensitivity to other drugs. Perhaps the most important criteria are that one exposure to a drug should not sensitize the patient to its subsequent administration and that the anaesthetic should release little or no histamine.

Sequelae

When propanidid was introduced, it was assumed that the high incidence of vomiting which followed its use for minor operations was due to the very rapid recovery. However, when it was found that this also occurred after ketamine, it was obvious that this explanation was too simple. Even allowing for the fact that a number of non-anaesthetic factors contributes to the occurrence of postoperative emesis, one would hesitate to recommend an induction agent which is followed by as high an incidence of sickness as either of these two drugs.

The emergence delirium which follows the use of ketamine, particularly in unpremedicated patients undergoing minor operations, is obviously undesirable. Similarly, unpleasant dreams and hallucinations are undesirable as they can affect a patient's attitude to subsequent anaesthetics.

While amnesia is a desirable property of small doses of an induction agent, the persistence of amnesia for a long time into the postoperative period is clearly undesirable. This effect should terminate with the return of consciousness, which should be smooth and pleasant.

One or more drugs?

From the above it will be apparent that there are a few properties which are essential for any ideal intravenous anaesthetic. Outside these there are others which are desirable but not essential (Table 12.3); if these cannot be achieved, then one may be prepared to accept different standards with respect to some actions.

We have two broad groups of myoneural blocking drugs with basically different pharmacological actions, durations of action and clinical uses. Within one of the groups we have a number of agents, the newer of which have been evolved to produce a drug which would be less toxic than the existing ones. Suxamethonium and one non-depolarizing blocker are essential for modern anaesthetic techniques and with these we can cover the complete span of clinical practice. Could this analogy be paralleled in the field of induction agents?

The barbiturates, eugenols and Althesin could be looked on as having the same basic action, with ketamine having a different mode of action. If the best features of the first three could be combined in one drug, this would give us a useful intravenous anaesthetic; it would be advantageous if this agent had a slight analgesic action and, perhaps, a central muscle relaxant action. This would be ideal not only for induction of anaesthesia but also as sole (or main) agent for minor procedures.

Table 12.3 Essential, desirable and acceptable properties for a new intravenous anaesthetic

Essential	Desirable	Acceptable
Physical properties as in Table 12.1	Adult anaesthetic dose in small volume	Volumes as for thiopentone
	Rapid onset Recovery from both redistribution and detoxication	Slight delay in onset
No antanalgesia	Slight analgesia	No analgesia
Smooth induction		Low incidence of mild complications
Good 'dose response' with respect to cardiovascular and respiratory effects	No dysrhythmias	
No myoneural blocking action		Slight muscular relaxation
No tendency to produce malignant hyperpyrexia	Cerebral metabolism and blood flow reduced	
Non-teratogenic	No histamine release	
Does not induce hypersensitivity on second exposure	Low incidence of hypersensitivity	
Low incidence of venous thrombosis	No effect on arterial injection	

For longer procedures a drug which features the physical properties, analgesia and duration of action of ketamine but without the same degree of cardiovascular stimulation and hypertonus and which is not followed by hallucinations or unpleasant dreams would be most useful. This would minimize the risk of awareness during anaesthesia, reduce the degree of theatre pollution from gases or vapours and possibly give a prolonged period of postoperative analgesia.

If anyone doubts the need for an 'ideal' anaesthetic agent or of more than one such agent, then the assessment of the present agents as set out in Table 12.4 should remove any doubts.

It has been said that the skill of the administrator is more important than the agent used. This is only partly true and no amount of experience can overcome some intrinsic drug disadvantages; perhaps the knowledgeable anaesthetist will avoid unsatisfactory agents in unsuitable patients. An ideal induction agent will not compensate for lack of knowledge, skill or experience by the administrator. However, if some of the obvious disadvantages of existing agents can be eliminated, then the ideal intravenous anaesthetic would make general anaesthesia a safe and more pleasant experience for patients. This, after all, is the objective not only of clinicians, research workers and teachers but also of this book.

Table 12.4 Assessment of the merit of available intravenous anaesthetics

	Thiopentone	Methohexitone	Propanidid	Althesin	Ketamine	Etomidate
Rapid onset	+	+	+	+	–	+
Recovery due to:						
redistribution	+	+		+	+	
detoxication		+	+	+		
Induction:						
Excitatory effects	–	+ +	+	+	+	+ + +
Respiratory complications	–	+	–	–	–	–
Cardiovascular: good dose response	+	+	–	+ +		+
Analgesic	–	–	+	±	+ +	–
Antanalgesic	+	+	–	–	–	?
Interaction with relaxants	–	–	+	–	–	–
Hypersensitivity not uncommon	–	–	+	+ +	–	–
Postoperative vomiting	–	–	+ +	–	+ +	
Emergence delirium	–	–	–	–	+ +	–

Index